Birth –
Through Children's Eyes

Sandra van Dam Anderson, R.N., M.S.

Doctoral Student in Nursing and Anthropology, University of Arizona College of Nursing

Nurse Educator in Community and Family Health Nursing

Co-Author of *Chronic Health Problems, Concept and Application* (Mosby, 1981)

Author of several journal articles, chapters, and reviews on the topic of Family-Centered Birth

and

Penny Simkin, R.P.T.

Childbirth Educator

Member, Editorial Board, *Birth and the Family Journal*

Author, co-author, or editor of a variety of books, pamphlets, and articles in the fields of childbearing and parenting.

110904

the pennypress
Seattle, 1981

This book is dedicated to my children: Josiah, who first made me wonder about birth through children's eyes, and Jana, whose birth was viewed with wonder by her brother.
—Sandra vanDam Anderson

To my family and to the hundreds of women and men who have been my students, from whom I have learned so much.
—Penny Simkin

Cover illustration by Marina Megale Horosko
Book designer: Daniel Kaylor

Printed in the United States of America

The Pennypress
1100 23rd Avenue East, Seattle, Washington 98112

Library of Congress Catalog Card Number: 81-82791
ISBN: 0-937604-05-4

CONTRIBUTORS

- **Lester Dessez Hazell**, M.A., C.R.C.

Faculty, Nurse Midwifery Education Program
University of California, San Francisco

Author of *Commonsense Childbirth, Birth Goes Home,* and a variety of articles and papers

- **Susan Parma**, R.N.

Childbirth Educator and Consultant
Maternity Nurse, Redwood Memorial Hospital, Fortuna, California

Previously, Initiator of the Sibling Preparation Program, Mt. Zion Hospital, San Francisco, California

Developed an Alternative Birthing Center at Peninsula Hospital, Burlingame, California

- **Paulina Perez**, R.N., B.S.N., A.C.C.E.

President of Childbirth & Family Education, Inc., providers of classes and workshops on the childbearing year, and continuing education workshops for health professionals.

Previously, Nurse Clinician and Director of Patient Education for a large obstetrical group in Houston.

- **Sara Pitta**, C.N.M.

Private Practice of Nurse-Midwifery

Childbirth Educator and Consultant in Family-Centered Maternity Care

Previously, Staff Nurse, Alternative Birthing Center, Mt. Zion Hospital, San Francisco, and teacher in the Sibling Preparation Program.

- ## Ann Armstrong Scarboro

Free-lance writer, mother of four children, two of whom born by cesarean section.

- ## David Stewart, Ph.D.

Executive Director, National Association of Parents and Professionals for Safe Alternatives in Childbirth

Author of *The Five Standards of Safe Childbearing*, co-editor of *Compulsory Hospitalization, Freedom of Choice in Childbirth?*, and numerous books and articles.

ACKNOWLEDGEMENTS

The authors and contributors would like to thank all of the children and parents who shared their experiences, enabling us to better understand children and birth.

In addition, Sandra Anderson wishes to thank Leta Brown Davis, R.N., and Laurie McCanless, R.N., for help in collecting and analyzing her data; and Eleanor Bauwens, R.N., Ph.D., Melinda Huie, R.N., and Margarita Kay, R.N., Ph.D., for reading manuscripts.

Penny Simkin wishes to thank Lola Caldwell for typing and retyping the manuscript.

Susan Parma and Sara Pitta wish to thank Doyle Buddington, David Sligar and their friends for their support and encouragement as their chapter was being written.

Paulina Perez wishes to thank her husband and three sons for their patience and understanding while she wrote her chapter; and Peter Thompson, M.D., and Leroy Leeds, M.D., for their open-mindedness in accepting the concept and for their continuing support of children at birth.

Ann Armstrong Scarboro wishes to thank her husband, James, for his support, Karen Garthe Moore, Dr. William J. Moore, Emily Jenkins-Reed for their encouragement, and Glenda Hiddessen for the use of her drawing of a cesarean birth.

TABLE OF CONTENTS

FOREWORD
LESTER DESSEZ HAZELL

The idea of having children present at birth has generated considerable heat and controversy, especially when birth takes place in a hospital. I am reminded that the same arguments were put forward about twenty years ago when the suitability of inviting the baby's father to be present was under question. Hospital personnel were concerned with whether the addition of the father would create more infection, upset the mother, and disrupt the whole birth process. Overriding all of these considerations, however, was the moral suitability of having the father present "at a time like that." Many obstetricians felt that it was inappropriate for husbands to witness the mother's nudity, and that their presence at the birth would mar their sex lives forever afterwards. Time has since proved the absurdity of making sweeping generalizations about what is or is not appropriate, and it is now accepted practice for the baby's father to be present if the mother so desires.

It is interesting to see the pattern repeated about the desirability of having children present for birth. When birth is to be at home, the question boils down simply to whom the mother wants to be present at her birthing. Friends and loved ones of any age who are able to contribute in positive ways are invited. Those who are discordant are not invited. No one postulates about negative effects on the children because of their ages. However, in the hospital, personnel are dealing with concerns of infection, disruption and morality in the same way they did for fathers.

It seems that what hospital personnel are really wrestling with has to do with their own uncertainty about how to fulfill their roles when children are present. Any unaccustomed newcomer creates anxiety. This has nothing to do with the merits to children of whether or not they witness a birth. However, it seems easier to raise concerns over the hazards to children or to the environment rather than to deal with the real issue, namely: how does a given hospital adjust to having children in unaccustomed places, and further, how does the staff deal with its feelings that it is morally wrong for children to be present at birth?

There is no question that children do require the environment to be structured differently than do adults. For example, very young children need someone with them to whom they relate comfortably, in order that their needs be met for food, rest and variety of experience. They also need someone to answer their questions and to explain. All children need to be able to move about and have a place to go when they get bored or tired or hungry. In return they get the opportunity to be helpful to the best of their ability in the process of getting another human being born. The personal rewards for doing this are as great for participating children as they are for anyone else. Children also contribute a fresh way of viewing what is happening and can enhance the experience for all concerned.

As for the moral question of whether children should or should not be present at birth, this seems to boil down to whether children should or should not experience all of life, whatever it brings, on their own terms. I see no evidence that children need to be shielded from either birth or death, and the attempts to do so create more problems than we realize at the time. Children can imagine all sorts of horrible, nightmarish creations in the absence of reality. Their imaginings are far worse than the most dire of reality because they have no facts on which to base their fears. Real fears can be dealt with and can be growth-producing. Nightmares remain in the world of fantasy.

Children develop very elaborate fears founded on the combination of adult fears and silence. Children fill in the gaps in their information with monster and goblin constructs. This is a very human trait. All through life our imaginings are far worse than the worst reality. Adult imaginings about the worst that can happen at birth and death set the scene for children to build even worse imaginings. They try to put into thought context the emotions and feelings that they pick up from the important adults in their lives. This is illustrated in many classic examples of children misconstruing the "facts of life" (note the euphemism, which sets the scene for misinformation in what it doesn't say). Children who are present for birth and death accept those realities and are afforded the opportunity to deal with their own growth as they expand their consciousness to take in wider experience. Whatever emotions arise can be integrated when they are based in reality.

For all of us, uncertainty, grief and mourning are a vital part of growth. They precede new integration at a higher level of experience. By restricting children's experiences we deprive them of the opportunity to take the reality of that experience and use it in ways appropriate to them.

Children are usually reasonably self-regulating when it comes to experiencing the birth process. They come and go at their own pace. I remember one birth in which a ten-year-old preferred to stay in the doorway while her five-year-old sister stayed on the bed the whole time. Obviously, the most important person during the labor is the mother, and her wishes and needs come first. Beyond that children do very well. I remember one birth at home in which the older brother and his best friend, both aged 2½ were asleep in the next room. As the baby crowned, they were awakened and brought in. Both clapped and watched enthralled as the baby emerged and took her first breath. Both touched the baby very gently with one finger. Then after it was clear that the process was pretty much over, one of them turned to the other and said, ''That's my little sister!'' The other one glared and said, ''No. She's not! She's mine!''

In another instance, a thirteen-year-old older-brother-to-be came in from playing baseball to find his mother in advanced first stage. He spent some time sizing up the situation, asked if it would be all right if he showered and then helped. He was back in ten minutes and spent the rest of the time giving his mother energy by being there quietly and meeting her eyes with his when she looked at him. He seemed to be saying to her: you and I went through this process together a long time ago and it worked out just fine. You can do it again now and it will be every bit as good. Her contractions became more efficient when he was there, and soon the baby was born. Big brother cut the cord under direction and along with the others there got acquainted with his new brother. After such a birth, the whole family gets to know and experience one another in many new and rewarding dimensions.

While the above examples were gleaned from my home birth experience, it is heartening to note that many alternative birth centers both in and out of hospitals are designed with children in mind. They provide space for children to munch, to rest, to play somewhat removed from where the mother is laboring. The supportive members of the family can stock the refrigerator with favorite edibles, cook on the stove, and a television, toys and books will go a long way in bridging time spans.

It is apparent to me that the only restrictions that need to be placed upon children's presence at birth are the desires of the mother and the logistical considerations discussed above. Attempts to shield children are misguided at the very least and can be a detrimental influence on the child for the rest of his life. In parallel, the same thing is true of death. As human beings, we are all responsible for assisting the comings-in and goings-out of our sisters and brothers regardless of our ages, each of us contributing at our own level of participation, whatever that is. Failure to do this creates the fabric for all sorts of non-participation in life based upon nameless fear and nightmare. When we live up to our responsibilities for birth and death, we experience and re-experience our Selves, our membership in that miracle that is humanity, and our oneness with all Creation in ever more meaningful levels of consciousness and being. The rewards are an increasing ability to go forth in this life with faith and confidence. We truly Know that birth and death are wondrous gateways for each of us.

1.

Children at Birth:
An Overview

SANDRA VAN DAM ANDERSON
and PENNY SIMKIN

Two discordant themes dominate today's attitudes toward childbearing, each claiming proponents and followers, each proceeding in its own direction. On the one hand is the theme that childbirth is always potentially hazardous, that a diagnosis of "normal" can only be made retrospectively, i.e., after the birth. Birth is so strange, mysterious, and dangerous that it must be controlled by experts, specialists and technicians. Presumably the experts are more able to produce a healthy baby than the physiological mechanisms of the human body.

This attitude results in a gradually increasing replacement of physiological labor mechanisms by artificial means to control parturition: e.g., the use of ultrasound, amniocentesis and other tests to determine the optimal date for delivery; the use of oxytocin, intravenous fluids, artificial rupture of the membranes, electronic fetal monitoring, analgesia, anesthesia, episiotomy, and forceps. Most conspicuous of all is the rapidly increasing use of cesarean section (approaching 15 to 25% in the United States) as the optimal mode of delivery. We have seen in the past decade, the development and institutionalization of a whole new medical subspecialty — perinatology. Through sophisticated technology, extended training of personnel, and development of neonatal intensive care nurseries, perinatologists exercise greater and greater control over the fetal-newborn period.

The second prevailing theme holds that most birth is normal and best conducted by relying on and enhancing the body's own physiologic mechanisms for parturition. The human female body is believed to be well-suited for giving birth and has finely tuned mechanisms (only a few of which are well-understood), for conception, pregnancy, birth and afterwards.

Management of childbearing is based on knowledge and participation by the parents, with the emphasis on health maintenance. Care is based on the principle of "watchful expectancy," that is, support and enhancement of the psychological and physiological process with the ability to recognize and act upon problems if they arise. Resulting from this attitude is an increase in practices such as: natural childbirth, psychological methods of pain relief, home births and birthing rooms in hospitals, attention to the emotional needs of families, breastfeeding, and attendance by midwives.

It is this trend which causes many parents to discard the idea that the birth of a child is something to be shrouded in mystery. A new openness of attitude toward family planning and childbearing has emerged in North America and other parts of the world over the past two decades. This openness has progressed to the point that some parents want to involve their children more in pregnancy and birth, even including them at the births of their siblings.

This chapter includes discussion of evolving patterns in birthing; ideas and feelings of adults and children about birth; cultural attitudes toward children at birth; sibling adjustments to a new baby; and objections or concerns raised against children attending birth.

TRENDS IN FAMILY-CENTERED BIRTHING

Parents and would-be parents have a wide range of educational material from which to choose in their attempts to educate themselves about pregnancy, birth and parenting. There is a wealth of material about childbirth preparation, pregnancy and birth, cesarean birth, home birth, breastfeeding, parenting and child development. There are special books for fathers, for children, for women over 30, and for teenagers. This explosion of educational material is also manifest in women's magazines, professional journals, and in materials available to childbirth educators. In addition to numerous films, videotapes, slide presentations, and models, there are also guides and manuals designed especially for childbirth education classes.

The approach to childbirth is indeed changing. It appears to be moving from the realm of privacy, modesty and mystery to a more public domain. This increasing openness about childbirth makes it possible to share the significant events associated with birth with those people who are dear to the childbearing family. Each birth is the birth of a new family unit; therefore, many people believe childbirth is an experience belonging to the entire family.

Who belongs to the childbearing family and deserves to participate at the birth? In the past this question was asked only in terms of who was allowed to visit the new mother on the postpartum unit. This person was usually the father. Perhaps he could catch a glimpse of his son or daughter in the nursery — if the shades were up and the crib was near the window. Older brothers and sisters of the newborn had little chance of seeing their mother, and were certainly not tolerated near the baby. Often the best arrangement that could be made was to wave to mother through the hospital window.

As the childbirth education movement, working to humanize the experience of labor and birth, gained momentum in the 1960's, new questions about family relationships and the roles of family members were asked. At that time it was assumed by many that fathers had little, if any, right or reason to be present during labor, and even less at birth. Surely, the father would contaminate the sterile field, be in the way, or faint. Due primarily to consumer demand, progress toward openness of birth as a family event continues. Fathers are present not only in birthing rooms and delivery rooms, but also at cesarean births in operating rooms.

The question of who belongs at a birth, and what role each plays is determined by the family alone when the birth takes place in the home setting. Such a choice is in contrast to hospital births, where the roles of "significant others" are determined by hospital policies and by the personal preferences of the obstetricians and nurses there at the time. The trend toward home births in the early 1970's was partly fueled by the desire of parents to determine who belongs to the childbearing family and what their roles would be at the birth. Inclusion of the whole family, even the children, at labor and birth is a natural decision for most people choosing a home birth. In fact, the desire to have a sibling present may be the major reason a couple chooses to have the birth at home.

Many hospitals have instituted a program of sibling visitation to accommodate those families who wish to include their children in welcoming the newborn and to minimize the trauma of separation from the mother. Some authors have investigated the role of siblings in the hospital. Rising (1974) stated there is a certain openness about the "fourth stage of labor" that may never occur again. Therefore, she advised visitation privileges as being essential for the newborn's siblings, if they are healthy. She proposed that sibling rivalry may be decreased if the children feel important enough to come to the hospital. Trause (1978) has found, however, that a one hour visit by the other child with the mother and new baby in the hospital is neither enough time to bring the two children close enough for attachment, nor to maintain attachment between the older child and the mother.

In a comparison study of women receiving traditional maternity care and family-centered care in a hospital, Jordan (1973) found that a high percentage of women in both groups stated they had desired to see their children during the hospitalization. Only the mothers in the family-centered care group, however, were allowed visits with their children. The majority of these mothers reported that the child's visit had relieved anxiety caused by separation of the mother and child. Many mothers in the traditional maternity care group stated that they felt alienated from their children, and anxious about their children's well-being while they were hospitalized. Jordan (1973) recommended that healthy children be allowed to visit their mother and the baby at least once during the hospitalization period.

Scaer and Korte (1978) interviewed 645 women by telephone to determine their preferences for 49 different options in maternity care. The most important area of concern was maintaining family closeness. More specifically, mothers wanted their other children to be able to see the new baby and to visit the mother during the hospital stay. Proposals resulting from this study included institution of family hours for sibling visitation with mother and baby, and development of hospital alternative birth rooms to accommodate family and friends for both labor and delivery.

Henson (1977) surveyed sibling visitation policies in 49 Arizona hospitals. Forty-five percent of the hospitals surveyed permitted sibling visitation in the halls or lounge. Only two hospitals permitted children in the mother's room. Fifty-five percent of the hospitals did not permit sibling visitation anywhere, except perhaps through a window. The usual explanation was that the hospital policy allowed no visitors under a certain age.

The American Academy of Pediatrics, however, has taken a different view on sibling visitation. The following statement appears in their *Standards and Recommendations for Hospital Care of Newborn Infants:*

> "Contact of a mother with her own family or special people is important after the birth of her infant. Moreover, her other children may need the reassurance of their mother's presence, however brief, after she has delivered. Therefore, visiting should not be restricted by the age of the visitor or the hour of the day." (American Academy of Pediatrics, 1977)

Some hospitals now permit parents to include their other children at the birth of a sibling in their "family-centered" birthing rooms. Many such facilities, however, while giving parents a wide range of options regarding their births, still, either by policy or by informal discouragement, do not allow or welcome children. A 1978 position statement by the Interprofessional Task Force on Health Care of Women and Children (including the American College of Obstetricians and Gynecologists, the American College of Nurse-Midwives, the Nurses' Association of the American College of Obstetricians and Gynecologists, the American Academy of Pediatrics, and the American Nurses' Association, and endorsed by the American Hospital Association) has influenced hospitals to rethink their policies in this area. The Task Force states that health care delivery should adhere to the following philosophy:

"— That the family is the basic unit of society;
— That the family is viewed as a whole unit within which each member is an individual enjoying recognition and entitled to consideration;
— That childbearing and childrearing are unique and important functions of the family;
— That childbearing is an experience that is appropriate and beneficial for the family to share as a unit;
— That childbearing is a developmental opportunity and/or a situational crisis, during which the family members benefit from the supporting solidarity of the family unit."

(Joint Position Statement on The Development of Family-Centered Maternity/Newborn Care in Hospitals, 1978)

The International Childbirth Education Association's 1978 *Position Paper on Planning Comprehensive Maternal and Newborn Services for the Childbearing Year* supports "presence of family and/or friends during labor, birth, and postpartum as desired by the childbearing woman." (ICEA, 1978).

Until all hospitals accept these position statements as their own policies, childbearing families will be dependent on the flexibility of individuals on hospital staffs for "bending" of the rules to include children. Personnel in some hospitals have quietly chosen not to enforce age visitation policies in either the postpartum or the labor and delivery rooms. In such situations, a family who wants to include children depends on the personnel and the availability of a room. This approach affords only minimal support to parents and children, either in preparation of children or at the birth itself.

ADULT ASSUMPTIONS ABOUT BIRTH

For some people, including many health professionals, the mere thought of children watching their mother give birth is enough to cause looks of disgust, expressions of outrage, and general reactions that suggest a sacred taboo is being broken. This group considers the idea of children at birth preposterous at best, probably illegal, and certainly immoral.

Most people have very definite opinions about the issue of siblings at childbirth. Clearly, the majority at first react against the idea. These opinions are usually based on their own adult "assumptions" about birth: that birth is painful, dangerous, frightening, unpleasant, private, mysterious, dirty, obscene. Some of these firmly-held opinions were printed in the newspaper column, "Dear Abby." It all began on March 3, 1980, with the headline, "Nothing Shocking in Witnessing Childbirth." A grandmother wrote that her daughter planned to have natural childbirth with the daughter's husband and three-year-old son present at the birth. This plan was contrary to the conservative modest background of the grandmother. Abby refused to be shocked, but suggested that witnessing childbirth might be the best way to learn about the miracle of life. That amazing answer brought a deluge of responses from readers across the country. The letters at one point were running 100-to-1 against her answer. Readers cynically suggested inviting little league teams and nursery school classes. One suggested it was child abuse. Several obstetrical nurses reacted strongly. One revealed her feelings that not only was there no need for hysterical kids, but hospital staffs could also do without the fainting fathers. There were some positive responses from convinced parents who indicated that presence at birth would help children be unafraid later, and would help them grow up respecting the miracle of birth.

In any community across the United States one is likely to hear these varied opinions expressed. Children's participation in childbirth is a new and controversial topic. The controversy implies that there is a right way and a wrong way to give birth. It is obvious, however, that sibling participation at birth is not for everyone. It need not be. It does need, however, to be an option that is available for consideration by expecting families. The practice of including siblings at childbirth can best be understood within the larger context of the alternative childbirth movement and the desire of many parents to share important experiences with children. Some parents believe childbirth belongs to the family as a whole. The *Birth Book* (Lang, 1972) has been used by many parents planning homebirths. This book was dedicated "to all children who will never have to ask, 'where do babies come from?' " (Lang, 1972).

CHILDREN'S IDEAS ABOUT BIRTH

Arnold Gesell once said that our knowledge of the child is about as reliable as a 15th century map of the world (Kellogg, and O'Dell, 1967). This statement certainly applies to our knowledge of children's ideas about the "facts of life" — sexuality, birth, and death. Adults often attempt to protect children from exposure to painful or puzzling information on these basic human functions, presumably on the assumption that they will be able to handle the information better when they become adults. Children, however, are exposed to birth, death, and sexuality through the media, conversations, pets, and day-to-day contact with their families and others. While we are just learning about children's perceptions of birth, we do know that children often do not share adults' distress concerning thoughts of death (Anthony, 1967). It is likely that children also have their own ideas about birth. These ideas may be somewhat vague and continually changing as children grow older and acquire experience. Perhaps adults should not assume that children share the prevailing adult attitude that birth is painful and unpleasant. Is it possible for adults to understand and learn from the vision of the child?

CULTURAL VARIATIONS ON CHILDREN AT BIRTH

The sociocultural meanings of birth and death vary widely from one society to another. Both birth and death cause changes in the social relationships of individuals and within kinship groups. These natural and biological processes of birth and death are woven into the cultural fabric of society. Ideas and beliefs about birth and death are emotionally embedded in each individual and family, in children and adults.

Cross-cultural literature indicates a broad range of cultural attitudes toward the involvement of children with childbirth. For some, birth is an open social event, while others surround it with secrecy. The Pukapuka from the Pacific Islands consider birth of interest to the whole community. Birth has no sense of mystery and is as natural as any other fact of life. A favorite game of the young children is to pretend cohabitation and simulate a pregnancy with a coconut under their clothes. After imitating labor pains, out falls the nut (Mead and Newton, 1967). Jarara women of South America give birth in full view of everyone, even small children (Newton and Newton, 1972). The Siriono Indians, who live in the tropical rain forest of eastern Bolivia, consider childbirth to be a public event. Childbirth normally takes place in a hut. The mother giving birth is well attended by women and children but rarely by the men. (Holmberg, 1969).

In contrast, other peoples feel the need for extreme privacy in birth. For instance, the Cuna of Panama do not permit children to see animals giving birth (Newton, 1974). Many societies avoid true explanations to children about sex and birth by telling them that specific animals or birds bring babies. Read (1968:23) reported that among the Ngoni of Malawi a "conspiracy of silence" about the origin of babies was maintained. Children are told that their mothers found the new baby on the river bank. Ngoni women explain the purpose of such an answer is to hide the secret of birth from the children and to discourage further questioning in order to follow cultural patterns of childhood innocence. Read noted, however, that in societies where this is the cultural approach to birth and sexual intercourse, "the stories were only standard replies to children, and most adults admitted that children pursued these inquiries among themselves and found out what they wanted to know from each other." In observations of the Nacirema (American) culture, Miner (1956) stated that parturition takes place in secret, without friends or relatives to assist.

In Western culture, most women gave birth at home until the 1940's, when the hospital replaced the home as the accepted site for birth. Before the shift to the hospital, it is unlikely that children were permitted to observe home births (Barker-Benfield, 1976). Even so, children were closer to the process at home than when births occurred in hospitals. Although there is no documentation of the role of children at early home births, oral history suggests that births were hidden from children and men to some extent. In most cases, women relatives, granny midwives, or doctors assisted with the birth while children watched the comings and goings of attendants. They probably tried to catch glimpses of the activities and heard unusual sounds. Their curiosity would have been soothed only after the birth, when they were welcome to see the baby.

As more and more women went to hospitals in the 1940's, they gave up control over the childbirth process to the physicians. The use of anesthesia and medication increased, resulting in intensive involvement in and further control by the physician. Active management of labor and delivery by the obstetrician has brought about many changes in birthing. Even though "medical management" can be beneficial when it is warranted, the routine use of technological interventions frequently causes a chain of events which distorts childbirth (Anderson, 1977).

The institutionalization of birth has resulted in dehumanization similar to that which has accompanied the institutionalization of death (Kubler-Ross, 1976). There are many parallels in our social attitudes toward the major life events of birth and death. Both tend to be mysterious, produce fear, and are generally very separate from daily living. Both birth and death are usually controlled by strangers and occur in unfamiliar territory. With both birth and death, however, there are movements to reclaim these events by families who wish to be supportive to one another, and to preserve individual dignity and personal choice.

The home birth movement is, in part, a response to the dehumanization of birth, as well as a desire by parents to include their other children in the birth process (Hazell, 1974).

SIBLING ADJUSTMENT TO A NEW BABY

Most people agree that becoming a sibling and adjusting to a new baby is a stressful situation for young children. Moore (1969) compared the sibling experience of a birth in the family with the uncommon childhood experience of parental death, claiming that both experiences have similar significance on later personality development. Legg (1974) reported that the younger the age at which the birth of a sibling is experienced, the greater the probability of disturbances. Overt negative reactions to the birth of a sibling were found in 89 percent of subjects under three years, while only 11 percent of children over six years showed this reaction. Sewell (1930) found that jealousy in the first sibling is likely when the second baby is born if the older child is between 18 and 42 months.

Many view pregnancy and childbirth as a "normal crisis," which has the potential for specific maturational gains for the entire family as a group, and for the individuals involved (Bibring, 1959). Mehl (1977) suggests, as a result of a study of 20 children present at births compared with 20 children not present, that the presence of children at a delivery permits an open attitude toward birth as a normal process in families where childbirth is accepted as normal. The children present tended to have very accurate notions about how babies are born, and seemed to view the birth in a positive manner. For girls, it aided in the development of their self-images as women. Less sibling rivalry among the children present was also suggested.

Chase (1976), after concluding her study of 55 home births in Salt Lake County, Utah, recommended the area of sibling rivalry for future research. Seventeen women (32%) chose a home birth because of a desire for more closeness of the mother, child, and the rest of the family. Eleven of the 55 women interviewed felt a home birth reduced the sibling rivalry in the families because their children had immediate contact with the newborns. Just as there is a sensitive period of maternal-infant attachment shortly after birth, perhaps there is also a sensitive attachment period between other members of the family and the newborn.

Curry (Maynard, 1977), a nurse-midwife who assists with home births, noticed that when a baby is born at home, the siblings associate the baby with rhythms of daily life, rather than with a frightening hospital where sick people go. She noted that when a mother goes to the hospital, the new baby is blamed for her disappearance; but when the children are present, the baby seems like a special gift. The presence of children at birth will probably not eliminate sibling rivalry, but parents report babies are easily integrated into family life when their coming has been a happy normal experience at home (Maynard, 1977).

In their book, Ward and Ward (1976) include sections written by parents about their experiences with home births. Many of these accounts state the parents' beliefs that the presence of siblings at a birth assures closeness between the siblings and the newborn from the very beginning of life. According to these parents, the older children feel no loss of love when they are allowed to be participants in this most important family event. Physicians who welcome children at birth have made similar observations. While they do not know the children nearly as well as the parents, their experiences with children at birth have raised no objections to the idea. Goodman (1976) noted no negative results from the inclusion of children in a hospital alternative birth room. Enkin (1976) believes there is much evidence that family attachment and closeness might be greatly enhanced by increased sibling involvement in childbirth. No regrettable experiences were encountered by Brew (Ward and Ward, 1976), who considers the presence of siblings at birth as purely an interesting episode in the lives of most children. Knapp (Ward and Ward, 1976), a nurse who assists with home births, was amazed at how well children manage at a birth. She has not seen any negative reactions, even with very young children, and believes the whole process is non-threatening to them. At times children have been concerned when watching their mothers in labor, but in her experience Knapp has observed that explanations given to the siblings present put the children at ease.

The Hathaways (1978) present a strong case for having children present at the births of siblings. Nevertheless, they do not recommend children's participation for all families. Negative parental feelings about birth and family modesty will certainly affect children's reactions. If children have not seen their mother nude, birth is probably not a good time to introduce them to her body. The Hathaways agree that children must be prepared in a manner that fits each individual child's age and developmental level.

One benefit of birthing at home is that siblings are not neglected. Other children in the family become part of the big event. Because the baby becomes their special present, "siblings are more accepting of the new little stranger" (Walker, et al, 1979). Is it possible that siblings experience bonding with their new brother or sister by a process similar to that which has been identified as maternal and paternal bonding? The two main authorities on the subject of maternal-infant bonding, Klaus and Kennell (1976), have identified basic principles in the process of attachment. One of these is that observers of the birth process become strongly attached to the infant. Lang (1972) also reports that witnesses of the labor and birth become more attached to the infant than do family and friends who were not present or who did not participate in the sensitive period immediately after birth. Kennell (1979) stated that there may be "great value to family solidarity in a positive home birth experience." But he expressed concern over possible long-term effects on children of different ages who witness childbirth. Montagu (1977) stated his belief that the early bond established between the father and his child would probably hold true for siblings were they allowed early contact with the newborn family member. This bond can possibly result in enduring beneficial effects upon siblings' relationships. Sonstegard (1976) commented that siblings need contact time with both parents and the new family member if they are to understand that they are not being deserted for another child. It is difficult for attachment to occur unless there is time to get acquainted. In the situation of a blended family (where both parents have children from previous marriages), it may be especially important for the family to share in the birth. The baby represents the common bond of all family members and can have particular significance in uniting the entire family.

Fragner (1979:33) believes that for children, bonding is a very different experience and serves a different purpose than for adults. "For children, the bonding process which begins to occur at birth is not rooted in biological necessity and serves a variety of emotional and social needs for each child. Children can use the sensitive period to begin examining the infant and discovering its unique traits; this exploratory experience serves as a bridge between the children's fantasy and the reality of the infant in their lives."

OBJECTIONS TO CHILDREN AT BIRTH

The desire of some parents to include children to some degree in birthing events has caused a negative reaction among health professionals. Many objections are based on concern for the welfare of the children, the emotional well-being of the mother, or worries about contamination and disruption of hospital procedures.

Pediatricians especially are concerned that the child may be emotionally traumatized by seeing the mother in pain, seeing the blood, the placenta, or the newborn. They are also worried over possible long-term negative effects. Some health professionals question whether the mother may feel pressured to be calm and quiet, whether she will be distracted by the presence of her child, or whether her partner will feel torn between supporting her and looking after the child. Nurses and physicians sometimes feel that "the delivery room is no place for children." Sterile technique may be broken. Children may play with delicate instruments, get in the way or generally create a disturbance in the hospital.

These concerns and objections disappear in those settings where a flexible family-centered attitude exists, when the children are well-prepared and have their own support person. In fact, many doctors, midwives and nurses have been pleasantly surprised by the spontaneous joy and air or normalcy that children bring to the birth.

In the only study of children attending hospital births, the authors found that during early labor children asked questions, timed contractions, and were solicitous of how the mother was feeling (Leonard, 1979). During late labor, only 3 children of 25 had to be removed (1 for being upset and 2 for being distracting). Most children took an observer role at this time. Of 33 children present at delivery, 31 watched, 1 hid his eyes, and 1 resisted being awakened. After the birth most children were engrossed with the baby and paid little attention to the delivery of the placenta. One child was upset when the mother required repair of the perineum. Children generally resumed normal activities soon after the birth, such as going to sleep if it was night time or having something to eat in the day time.

As the authors state: "Children watch the process, attend to the infant, and then are quickly ready to resume their regular activities." While many would conclude from the data that children take birth readily in stride, the authors surprisingly concluded that, "Childbirth is primarily an adult event," presumably because the children's excitement was of shorter duration than the parents.

As Leonard, et al., point out, "When children are present, it appears to be a wish of their parents that they be there." This raises an interesting question about the motivation of parents who choose to include their children at birth. Fragner (1979) found that conscious motivation to include children at birth seems to stem from a strong commitment to the family structure, and from a perception of childbirth as a natural healthy family event. She believes that families who choose to include children value direct and matter-of-fact communication about sexual matters and view the birth of a baby as part of that communication process.

Complex and unconscious feelings may also motivate parents to include children at birth: cultural and social pressures to portray an avant-garde lifestyle; need for support from their children; unresolved sexual issues between mother and child; fears of parents about birth and sexuality (Fragner, 1979).

Some detractors object that having children attend births teaches them too much about sex too soon. The question is cynically asked, "Why not have them present at conception?" as if the next logical step after opening birth to the eyes of children is to include them in observation of sexual intercourse. At first glance this may seem to be a valid objection, but the issue deserves a closer look. Intercourse and birth, although connected physiologically, are not comparable in their significance or impact on each family member. Sexual intercourse is a private personal matter with little or no effect on anyone except the couple involved, while the birth of a baby permanently alters the lives of all family members and, to a lesser extent, all of society.

The appropriate age of children is also a matter of uncertainty. Some have expressed the opinion that teenagers are too caught up in their own struggle for sexual identity to comfortably experience birth. Others believe that children under four years of age are unable to understand birth and, because they are dependent on their mothers for emotional support, they should be discouraged from attending birth (Leonard, 1979).

Does a child have to understand birth in an adult way in order to benefit from the experience? It may be that children who are close to and dependent on their mothers should not be separated during this significant change in the family. Therefore, the issue of whether some ages are more appropriate than others continues to be raised. At this point there is no evidence that birth is any less positive for children of one age than of another. It is likely that children of various ages absorb from the birth experience at a level compatible with their age and development.

As for the concern about contamination or increased danger of infection for the newborn or other newborns, hospitals can adopt protocols which provide safeguards against infection by the older child. Siblings should be screened for illness before attending a birth. Children with fevers, runny noses, coughs, or other symptoms of illness can be asked to stay at home. Children can be expected to scrub and gown before holding the newborn. In addition, they can be restricted to appropriate areas of the hospital only: the birthing room and all "public" areas. The child can be expected to have contact only with his/her own newborn sibling. The newborn usually stays with the family until discharge, but even if returned to the nursery, if the above precautions have been observed, the newborn is no more likely to bring infection into the nursery after contact with a sibling than after contact with the father. If the hospital staff fears that a newborn who has been handled by his/her sibling will spread infection in the nursery, the newborn can be kept in isolation. In those hospitals experienced with siblings attending births and/or sibling visitation, the fear of infection has declined as they have observed good results.

CONCLUSION

Many parents are demanding more choices in the realm of childbirth, and more input into the decisions about the births of their children. The choice of whether to include siblings at the birth has many issues involved: cultural taboos; feelings and ideas of parents and professionals about birth; children's feelings and ideas about birth; family desires; readiness and age of children; motivation of parents; sibling attachment, and many others.

Regardless of the objections, some parents are choosing to include children at birth. Therefore, it is important to continue to study the many issues and questions being raised by parents and professionals.

REFERENCES

American Academy of Pediatrics. *Standards and Recommendations for Hospital Care of Newborn Infants.* 6th Edition, 1977.

Anderson, S.F., "Childbirth as a pathological process: an American perspective." *The American Journal of Maternal Child Nursing* 2(4): 240-244, July-August, 1977.

Anthony, S., "The child's idea of death," in Talbot, T. (ed.), *The World of the Child.* New York: Doubleday and Company, Inc., 1967.

Barker-Benfield, G.J., *The Horrors of the Half-Known Life.* New York: Harper and Row, 1976.

Bibring, G.L., "Some considerations of the psychological processes in pregnancy," in Eissler, R. (ed.), *Psychoanalytic Study of the Child.* New York: International Universities Press, 1959.

Chase, E., "Home births in Salt Lake City in 1975." Master's thesis, University of Utah College of Nursing, 1976.

Enkin, M., "The family in labour." *Birth and the Family Journal,* 2 (4): 133-136, 1975-6.

Fragner, R.B., "A model for examining the psychological implications of children's participation in birth." Doctoral dissertation, California School of Professional Psychology, Berkeley, CA: 1979.

Goodell, R., "Bringing up the children by taking them to birth." *New York Times,* Feb. 24, 1980, p. E9.

Goodman, M., "Experiences with a labor/delivery room." *Birth and the Family Journal* 3: 123, Fall, 1976.

Hathaway, M. & Hathaway, J., *Children at Birth.* Sherman Oaks, CA: Academy Publications, 1978.

Hazell, L.D., *Birth Goes Home.* Seattle: Catalyst Press, 1974.

Henson, D., Report: *Hospital resources related to alternatives in maternity care in Arizona,* 1977.

Holmberg, A.R., *Nomads of the Long Bow: The Siriono of Eastern Bolivia.* Garden City, NY: The Natural History Press, 1969.

International Childbirth Education Association, *Position Paper on Planning Comprehensive Maternal and Newborn Services for the Childbearing Year.* Minneapolis, MN: 1978.

Interprofessional Task Force on Health Care of Women & Children, *Joint Position Statement on the Development of Family-Centered Maternity/Newborn Care.* Chicago, IL: 1978.

Jordan, D., "Evaluation of a family-centered maternity care hospital program." *Journal of Obstetric, Gynecologic, and Neonatal Nursing* 2 (1): 15-22, 1973.

Kellogg, R. and O'Dell, *The Psychology of Children's Art.* New York: CRM-Random House, 1967.

Kennell, J.H., Personal Communication, 1979.

Klaus, M.H. & Kennell, J.H., *Maternal-infant Bonding.* St. Louis: C.V. Mosby, 1976.

Kubler-Ross, E., *Death: The Final Stage of Growth.* New York: Harper and Row, 1976.

Lang, R., *Birth Book.* Fulton, CA: Genesis Press, 1972.

Legg, C. et al., "Reaction of preschool children to the birth of sibling." *Child Psychiatry and Human Development* 5 (1): 3-29, 1974.

Leonard, C.H., "Preliminary observations on the behavior of children present at the birth of a sibling." *Pediatrics* 64 (6): 949-951, December, 1979.

Maynard, F., "Home births vs. hospital births." *Women's Day,* June 28, 1977, pp. 10, 12, 161-164.

Mead, M., and Newton, N., "Cultural patterning of perinatal behavior." In Richardson, S.A. and Guttmacher, A.F. (Eds.). *Childbearing: Its Social and Psychological Aspects.* Baltimore: Williams and Wilkins, 1967.

Mehl, L.E., Brandsel, C. and Peterson, G.H., "Children at birth: effects and implications." *Journal of Sex and Marital Therapy* 3 (4): 274-279, 1977.

Miner, H., "Body ritual among the Nacirema." *American Anthropologist,* LVIII, 1956: 503-507.

Montagu, A., "Social impacts of unnecessary intervention and unnatural surroundings in childbirth," in Stewart, D. and Stewart, L. (ed.) *21st Century Obstetrics Now.* Chapel Hill, NC: NAPSAC Publication, 1977.

Moore, T., "Stress in Normal Childhood." *Human Relations* 22:3, 1969.

Newton, N. and Newton, M., "Childbirth in cross-cultural perspective," in Howells, J.G., (ed.). *Modern Perspectives in Psycho-Obstetric* (No. 5). New York: Brunner-Mazel Publishers, 1972.

Newton, N., "Some aspects of primitive childbirth." *Journal of the American Medical Association,* June 8, 1964, 188, 261-264.

Parma, S., "A family-centered event? Preparing the child for sharing in the experience of childbirth." *Journal of Nurse-Midwifery* 24 (3): 5-10, 1979.

Perez, P., "Nurturing children who attend the birth of a sibling." *American Journal of Maternal Child Nursing* 4: 215-217, 1979.

Read, M., *Children of Their Fathers: Growing Up among the Ngoni at Malawi.* New York: Holt, Rinehart and Winston, 1968.

Rising, S., "The fourth stage of labor: family integration." *American Journal of Nursing* 74 (5): 870-874, 1974.

Scaer, R. and Korte, D., "MOM survey: maternity options for mothers — what do women want in maternity care?" *Birth and the Family Journal* 5 (1): 20-26, 1978.

Sewell, M., "Some causes of jealousy in young children." *Study of Social Work* 1: 23-40, 1930.

Sonstegard, L., "Family-centered nursing makes a difference." *American Journal of Maternal Child Nursing* 1 (4): 249-254, 1976.

Trause, M., "Birth in the hospital: the effect on the sibling." *Birth and the Family Journal* 5 (4): 207-210, Winter, 1980.

Walker, M., Yoffe, B. and Gray, P., *The Complete Book of Birth.* New York: Simon and Schuster, 1979.

Ward, F., & Ward, C., *The Home Birth Book.* Washington, D.C.: Inscape Press, 1976.

2.

Comparison Study of Children Present and Absent at Birth of Siblings*

SANDRA VAN DAM ANDERSON

What about children at birth? This question is being asked by parents, children, childbirth educators, nurses, midwives, obstetricians and pediatricians. Almost everyone has a very definite answer to that question. The answers range from, "Absolutely yes, children are members of the family and belong at the birth event," to "Positively no." In the words of a pediatrician: "It could scare the daylights out of a kid. And preparing a child for what he would see during the birth would not make a difference. You can't prepare a six-year-old. Hell, they don't know what's going on." (Stengel, 1979). It seemed to me that many opinions on this sensitive issue were based on very little knowledge of children at birth and little or no direct experience with children at birth. I was aware of positive anecdotes, but found a void in the professional literature on this subject. This motivated me to design an exploratory comparison study.

The purpose of this study was to learn about the responses of siblings to pregnancy, birth and the newborn, as perceived by the parents. The goals were to identify possible concerns of children during labor and birth; to prepare guidelines for preparation of "expecting" siblings; and to suggest policies for birthing rooms and for hospital visitation for siblings.

DESCRIPTION OF STUDY

An interview protocol was developed to focus on four areas: 1) family

---

*This chapter is adapted from "A Scientific Survey of Siblings at Birth," by Sandra Anderson, R.N., M.S., and Leta J. Brown, R.N., C.C.E., in *Compulsory Hospitalization or Freedom of Choice in Childbirth*, vol. 3 (Marble Hill: NAPSAC, 1979). Available from NAPSAC, P.O. Box 267, Marble Hill, MO 63764.

activities in preparation for a baby, 2) the reaction of a child at the birth, 3) the reaction of the child to the infant and parents, and 4) the long-term relationship of the child and infant (Appendix A). Twenty-five families who had a home birth with a total of 43 children present were interviewed in their home setting. Usually the mother was the main source of information; however, children were often present and added information when they started to feel comfortable with the interviewers. Fathers were also present on occasion, and contributed to the answers. Most of the families were contacted through the Arizona School of Midwifery in Tucson, Arizona. Midwives trained at this school had assisted at many of the home births where siblings were present.

A comparison sample population of 25 families was also interviewed. These families consisted of parents, with a total of 39 children, who recently had a baby born in the hospital without siblings present. The same interview protocol was used with minor variations in the section concerning children present at the birth. These families were reached through instructors of both Bradley and Lamaze Childbirth Preparation classes. The study populations were chosen because of anticipated similarities; however, the quantity and complexity of variables were recognized. Legg (1974) was aware of the many variables that enter into a study of the reaction to sibling birth when the mother is hospitalized: separation from the mother, increase or decrease of father involvement with the child, different caretaker, and even a possible change of living quarters. It was inevitable that each child's situation would be unique in many ways.

DESCRIPTION OF POPULATION

The two study populations, one having home births with siblings present, and the other having hospital births without siblings present, were selected from settings where the demographic data were anticipated to be similar in terms of family structure, ethnic group, age, educational level, occupation, and religious affiliation. Demographic data were collected in order to present a profile of the populations with siblings present and without siblings present (Table 1). In the population with siblings present, the maternal age ranged from 20 to 37 years, a mean of 28.6 years. The paternal age range was from 23 to 41 years. Education of the mothers ranged from 10 to 18 years, with 15 of the 25 having more than a high school education. The fathers' education ranged from 11 to 21 years, with 17 of 25 having more than a high school education.

TABLE 1:
DEMOGRAPHIC CHARACTERISTICS OF POPULATIONS
WITH SIBLINGS PRESENT AND ABSENT AT BIRTH.

	Siblings Present	*Siblings Absent*
Mother's mean age	28.6 years	27.6 years
Father's mean age	31.0	28.7
Mother's mean years of education	14.1	13.5
Father's mean years of education	14.8	14.3
Sibling's mean age	4.7	5.4

In comparison, the population without siblings present represented a maternal age range from 23 to 36 years. The fathers ranged in age from 25 to 40 years. Education of the mothers ranged from 11 to 16 years, with 15 of 25 having more than a high school education. The fathers' education ranged from 9 to 19 years, with 20 of 25 having more than a high school education.

All 50 families had a traditional nuclear family structure with mother, father and children in the home. All of the subjects were Caucasian in the group with siblings present. This included two parents who were of Mexican ancestry. The group without siblings present were, also, all Caucasian, with six mothers and five fathers of Mexican ancestry.

The group with siblings present included 16 of 25 mothers who identified themselves as housewives, homemakers, home engineers, or managers, as compared with seventeen in the homemaker category of the population with siblings absent (Table 2). Mothers who held professional or white collar jobs were typically employed as teachers, counselors, and nurses. Skilled workers included secretaries and cashiers. Fathers employed as blue collar workers or craftsmen included metal workers, janitors, cabinet makers, painters, groundsmen, carpenters, mechanics, and miners. Professional or white collar fathers were mainly teachers, engineers, salesmen, administrators, and ministers.

The religious profile of the group with children present yielded 13 families who were active in a church, and 12 families who were either inactive or identified no religion for themselves. In comparison, the group with children absent at birth yielded 20 families who were active in a church, and five families who were inactive.

The ages of the children present at a birth ranged from 2 to 16 years, with a mean of 4.7 years. There were 36 children in the age range from 2 to 6 years. In comparison, the 39 children who were not present at a birth ranged in age from 1 to 13 years, with a mean of 5.4 years. Twenty-five children were in the range from 2 to 6 years (Figure 1).

TABLE 2:
OCCUPATIONAL CHARACTERISTICS OF POPULATIONS WITH SIBLINGS PRESENT AND ABSENT AT BIRTH.

	Siblings Present	Siblings Absent
Mother's Occupation		
Homemaker	16	17
Professional/white collar	8	5
Skilled	0	3
Student	1	0
Father's Occupation		
Blue collar/craft	10	12
Professional/white collar	11	12
Student	2	1
Unemployed/disabled	2	0

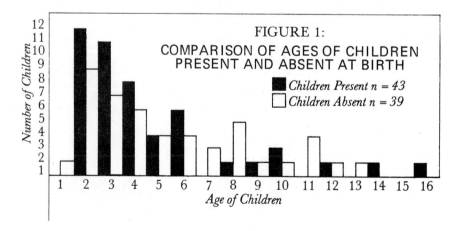

FIGURE 1:
COMPARISON OF AGES OF CHILDREN PRESENT AND ABSENT AT BIRTH

Children Present n = 43
Children Absent n = 39

Number of Children

Age of Children

RESULTS OF STUDY

The first set of questions focused on family activities in preparation for the baby. All of the results will be reported by family, with exceptions noted, because usually all children within a family participated in a similar fashion. All of the 50 families in both groups of the study population brought the children into discussions about the baby at various times. In the group with siblings present at birth, four families included the children in the idea of expanding the family, even before conception. Eighteen families told the children about the pregnancy as soon as it was confirmed; three families

---

TABLE 3:

TIME FRAME WHEN CHILDREN PRESENT AND ABSENT AT BIRTH WERE TOLD ABOUT BABY.

	Families with Children Present	Families with Children Absent
	n = 25	n = 25
Before conception	4	1
When pregnancy confirmed	18	16
When pregnancy "showed"	3	8

---

shared the information with their children when the mother displayed obvious physical signs of pregnancy (Table 3).

In the group without siblings present at a birth, one couple told their children about the plan to have a baby before conception; sixteen families communicated the news to the children at the time the pregnancy was confirmed; and eight families first shared the information when the pregnancy "showed."

All of the families in both of the groups showed the children pictures of fetuses, let the children try using the things for the baby, such as diapers, bottle, and crib. Many of the children either had a doll or got one in relation to the arrival of the baby.

During the prenatal period, all of the families with children present and all of the families without children present except one let the children frequently feel the fetus move in the mother's abdomen. The reactions of the children were described as follows: excited, giggled, thrilled, amazed.

Twenty of the 25 families with children present at birth included the children in prenatal care by taking them to the doctor's or midwife's office (Table 4). This activity usually stimulated questions, giving the child an opportunity to become acquainted with the doctor or midwife, as well as medical instruments. This event was reported as enjoyable for the child. Children who had a chance to hear the fetal heart beat by way of the ultrasound stethoscope were excited, and were described as smiling and glowing. If an ultrasound stethoscope was not available, children enjoyed using the fetoscope, but usually were unable to hear fetal heart tones. It was reported that all health care givers for this group were open to children being present at the prenatal visits, and encouraged participation by the children.

In contrast, of the 25 families without children present, 12 families included the children by taking them to one or more prenatal visit, and by allowing them to be with the mother. An additional two families took the children to the doctor's office, but the children were not allowed in the examining room. The children were thus able to meet the doctor and ask questions. Three families brought the children along for the prenatal visit, but the children were left in the waiting room where they had no interaction with the staff. Eight families did not include the children in any prenatal visits, which was usually explained by the mother as due to her discomfort in having the children present, no opportunity to include the children, didn't think of it, because the doctor wouldn't allow children in the examining room, or they were afraid to ask the doctor. Fourteen of the families in the group without children present allowed children to listen to fetal heart

TABLE 4:

LEVEL OF PARTICIPATION IN PRENATAL CARE SETTING BY CHILDREN PRESENT AND ABSENT AT BIRTH.

	Families with Children Present	Families with Children Absent
	n = 25	n = 25
In examining room	20	12
In examining room except for pelvic exam	0	2
In waiting room	0	3
Not included in prenatal care	5	8

sounds. Eleven families did not provide this experience, usually because of lack of opportunity.

All of the parents in both groups said they were willing to answer questions about childbirth asked by their children. Fifteen of the 25 families with children present recalled that questions were in fact asked. The three to six-year-old children were most likely to ask questions, and their most common question was, ''How will the baby get out?'' Parents reported that the older children didn't ask questions because they already knew the answers. However, one ten-year-old was wondering, ''How many times to you have to do it before you get pregnant?''

TABLE 5:
PARTICIPATION IN CHILDBIRTH PREPARATION CLASSES BY CHILDREN PRESENT AND ABSENT AT BIRTH.

	Families with Children Present	Families with Children Absent
	n = 25	n = 25
Midwives' classes	13	0
Bradley classes	4	4
Lamaze classes	0	1
No classes	8	20

Childbirth preparation classes were attended by 22 families in the group without children present at birth. Fourteen couples attended classes teaching the Bradley method, and eight couples attended Lamaze classes. Out of 25 families, five brought their children along to the preparation classes.

In the group without children present, 16 families remembered that children actually asked questions. Again, children in the age range from three to six were most likely to ask questions. And, as with the other group, the most common question was regarding the baby ''getting out'' of the mother. One five-year-old was certain the baby would have to be cut out. Explanations with pictures did not help, according to the mother. A four-year-old was puzzled how the baby could be small enough to come out of the ''belly button.'' An eight and a twelve-year-old used the opportunity of pregnancy to validate information they already had. Children younger than three years old in both groups seldom asked any questions.

All of the couples having a home birth with children present attended childbirth preparation classes. Seventeen of the 25 couples brought their children along to one or more of the childbirth preparation classes. Thirteen of those couples attended parent education classes given by trained midwives at the Arizona School of Midwifery, and four couples took their children to Bradley classes (Table 5). Responses of children to the classes ranged from "interested" to "played with other kids" to "slept." One mother said that her child seemed to pay no attention, but at the time of birth her daughter recognized the midwives and the birth chair, as well as the function of each.

Children from 16 families from the group with the children present saw either a film or television program portraying a birth. Some of the children saw the television program, "My Mom's Having a Baby." Children in a family who had witnessed a home birth were shocked by the conditions in the hospital, and reacted negatively to the "unfriendly" environment. Most of the children attending classes by midwives saw a film of a home birth. Some of the reported reactions are listed below:

> Very interested and intent.
> Watched the birth itself — ran around the rest of the time.
> Thought the baby looked "yucky."
> Commented on noises made by mother during labor.
> Thought it strange the way the baby came out.
> Excited about the baby being "brand new."
> Very blase.
> Thought it was messy, and thought the placenta was "gross."
> Enthusiastic.
> Fascinated.

Children in 14 families in the group not present at birth saw the television program, "My Mom's Having a Baby." Most of the children were reported as being interested, and some were perceived as being surprised. Four families took their children to see the Bradley childbirth film, "Childbirth for the Joy of It."

The second area of questioning dealt with the perceived reaction of the children during labor and birth. We were interested in the location of the children who were present at birth, which most parents left up to the children themselves. In general, the children continued with their activity as usual. Ten of the children slept during some part of the labor or birth. The children were in and out of the birth room, some staying near the mother at times and others playing in another room or outside. One child refused to leave the house and go to the neighbors, as planned. In another family the three children were kept out of the bedroom during pelvic exams and during the birth, but they stayed right outside the door, peeked in as often as possible, and came in before the cord was actually cut. The mother had no clothes on, which was a big surprise to the children, as they had never seen her that way before. This was a major reason why she did not want the children present at the birth. Another child was at home for the early stages of labor, but was picked up, as prearranged, by relatives and taken to their home. The child protested strongly by crying and ''having a fit,'' because she desperately wanted to stay at home. She seemed to realize that an important event was going to happen.

Children in five families in the group of siblings not present at birth were in the hospital waiting room during the birth. Nine families had grandparents with the children and eleven families used neighbors, relatives, friends, and sitters to care for the children during the birth.

We also asked who related to the children during labor and birth. In ten families, the father was the primary person relating to the child, although other fathers expressed being too busy and preoccupied with the mother to be able to concentrate on the child. Nine families had arranged for an additional person to come specifically to care for and relate to the children. This person was usually a friend, grandparent, or teacher of the child. In six families, the mother was the primary person relating to the child. Some mothers made every effort to talk with their children between contractions. However, other mothers verbalized a need not to be distracted by children during the labor and birth. Some children participated directly by bringing ice chips or cold cloths, and one older child helped the mother walk during labor.

The overall reactions of the children present at labor and birth were considered by the researchers to be positive without qualification in 22 of 25 families. These children were perceived to be curious, calm, supportive, and excited. One youngster reacted to a groan from the mother as the head was crowning, and the father was preparing to catch the baby, by patting the mother lovingly saying, ''It's okay, daddy won't do it again.'' Two children were considered to have a qualified positive experience. One event in this category involved a two-year-old who was awakened in the middle of the night for the birth. The child cried softly for a brief period and clung to the father. However, older children who were awakened for the birth or stayed up late were very pleased and proud to participate, even in the middle of the night. The second qualified positive experience involved a three-year-old who was shocked at the blood, and decided the mother and baby were both dead. This naturally scared the child, but because of the discussions which followed, the parents considered it a positive learning experience for the child. The one negative experience involved the three-year-old who was present for the labor, but was removed from the home against her will before the birth of the baby.

The reaction of the children present at the birth to the newborn sibling in 17 of 25 families was to reach out and touch the baby. Six children immediately offered a special present, such as a rattle or one of their dolls or toys, to the new brother or sister. Some of the children helped wrap the infant in blankets and held the baby. Two children were openly protective of the infant. One child told the midwives as they were packing up the equipment: "Don't take my baby." Another child was upset with the pediatrician who came to the home to do a newborn assessment. The four-year-old protested as the doctor examined the eyes with a bright light, and tested the reflexes. One six-year-old boy was disappointed to have a sister, and ignored her the first day.

Of the 39 siblings not present at birth, 26 of them visited the hospital following the birth. One two-year-old who frequently asked, "Where's mommy?" was not taken to see her mother because the parents were afraid that she would be too upset when visiting hours were over. Likewise, the mother did not talk with her on the phone for fear of triggering an unpleasant reaction. Most of the children saw their mothers in the lobby. A five-year-old was very concerned to see his mother in a wheel chair. Several children observed, and seemed surprised, that their mothers were "not fat anymore." A two-year-old and a four-year-old cried after visitation because they didn't want to leave their mothers and new siblings in the hospital. A child whose mother had a cesarean birth was not allowed to see either his mother or his new sibling for five days. Most of the children viewed their new siblings through a window from a distance. One child wondered how such a big baby could possibly have been inside of the mother. One eight-year-old girl, who informed her mother that she did not like to see her "fat," i.e., pregnant, and that she did not want her to get pregnant again, was convinced that childbirth is very painful. She did not want to hear about the birth; however, when she saw her baby sister for the first time, she thought she was beautiful, and has been accepting of her since the first view. One hospital sends birth cards home with the fathers for the siblings. The nurse wrote in a personalized message for each sibling and signed it with the baby's foot print.

I also gathered data about the reactions of the siblings to the infants in the weeks and months following the birth (Table 6). Of the 43 children present at the birth of a sibling, 42 wanted to participate in the care of the infant. Thirty-eight of the 39 siblings not present at the birth also wanted to participate in the care of the baby.

TABLE 6:

BEHAVIORS OF SIBLINGS TOWARD INFANTS BY SIBLINGS PRESENT AND ABSENT AT BIRTH.

	Siblings Present n = 43		Siblings Absent n = 39	
	Frequency	Percent	Frequency	Percent
Participate in care	42	98%	38	97%
Regressive behavior	8	19%	13	33%
Abusive to infant	7	16%	13	33%

Regressive behavior was noted in eight (19%) of the 43 children present at the birth of a sibling, and in 13 (33%) of 39 children not present at the birth. Return to daytime wetting was noted most frequently in recently toilet-trained two- and three-year-olds. Other regressive behavior noted was the return to thumb sucking, baby talk, nighttime wetting, and stuttering.

Abusive behavior was identified in seven (16%) of the 43 children present at birth, and in 13 (33%) children not present. Abusive behavior included pinching, hitting the baby or parents, trying to push the baby off the parent's lap, and intentionally hugging too tightly.

I also asked if children wanted to try milk from a bottle or breast. Out of 43 children who were present at birth, 13 wanted to try breast milk, and all were satisfied after one taste. One child wanted to try a bottle. Of the 39 siblings not present at birth, six wanted to try breast milk and two wanted to try the bottle.

I questioned parents about their relationship with the children fol-lowing the birth. Nine parents from the group with children present at birth reported that they were closer to the children; six stated that the children were closer than usual to the father in the first week following birth; six said the relationships stayed the same, and behavior problems were experienced in four families. In families where children were not present at the birth, eight parents felt that they were closer to the children; three thought the children related to the father more than usual; four families thought the relationships stayed the same. Ten of the parents reported some problem in their relationship to their children; for instance, unruly behavior, possessiveness, and whining to get attention.

Of the 43 siblings present at a birth, all of them were perceived by the parents as being very close to the infant in the first weeks. However, in the families in both study groups where the infant was at least one year old, some of the siblings were fighting with the baby, which seemed to begin when the baby became mobile, and started to bother them. Of the 39 siblings not present at birth, 24 were perceived as having loving relationships with the new sibling, 10 were indifferent, and five were jealous.

Parents were asked, "Do your children see you undressed?" Seventeen of 25 couples who had children present at the birth were frequently nude around the children in the house. Seven couples were undressed occasionally around the children, such as in the bathroom or getting dressed or undressed. One couple described their whole family as very modest, and the parents were never seen undressed by the children. In the group of parents without children present, 15 parents stated they were frequently nude around the house, six couples were occasionally undressed around the children, and four parents claimed they were never undressed around the children.

The last question asked was: "Is there anything you wish had happened differently in regard to your child or children participating in the pregnancy and birth?" Some of the comments from the families whose siblings were present are listed:

My child woke up as the baby's head was coming out. I would have liked her there about 20 minutes earlier.

Sorry the child cried when awakened, but not sorry we woke her.

I wish I didn't have to go to the hospital due to the placenta accreta. Then my child wasn't allowed in hospital, and wondered what was wrong.

We would not have given so much special attention to the three-year-old, which made her wonder "what's going on." When the excitement and visitors wore down, she noticed the lack of attention and was very jealous.

Our children went to friends for a few days following the birth. Wish we would have kept them at home. The two-year-old cried when he left, and acted hurt when he came home by sitting with the friend instead of sitting with me.

I would have encouraged my child to be on the bed in order to get a better view of the birth.

I wish my child had been awake, but that's okay. I plan to have more.

I wish that we had prepared the kids specifically about the blood. They saw books and movies in black and white, but that wasn't sufficient. Births are in living color.

I would have liked a vaginal birth with my son present instead of a cesarean birth.

If the kids wanted to be there, I would want them there.

I would have had my children closer together and at home.

I wish I had been brave enough to ask the doctor if my child could have gone to the prenatal exams, especially to hear the heartbeat.

I wouldn't have worked as a registered nurse in an intensive care nursery which caused undue anxiety.

I was overly involved with breastfeeding, and uptight with my two-year-old.

Several families mentioned that they wished they had taken more pictures, or had one person especially assigned to do photography. At the time of birth it didn't seem important because everyone was sure the event would be unforgettable. Some people thought the picture-taking would be distracting. However, mothers seemed to appreciate the pictures the most. Perhaps that is one way a mother can fill in the "missing pieces" (Affonso, 1978), and reconstruct the events surrounding the birth when she was focused on bringing the baby into the world.

Families whose children were not present at the birth were also asked if, with hindsight, they would have liked anything different. Four mothers said they would have liked to have had their children present. Following are some of the comments:

Three families wished that they had taken their children to the hospital for contact with the mother and new baby. One mother wanted to tell her daughter, who was in school at the time, about the birth, but the neighbor who picked up the child beat her to it.

DISCUSSION

In spite of the existing taboo on open childbirth, siblings are being included at births. Children are accepting this maturing experience with an overwhelmingly positive reaction. Parents feel there are many benefits in having their other children present, as it truly makes both the pregnancy and birth a family affair.

The learning potential for children is very high when their mother is pregnant. Many people are excited about this potential when pets are pregnant and give birth. However, the growth-producing experience that is possible when a mother is pregnant is often overlooked. It is an excellent time for children to learn about human bodies, sexuality, conception, life and growth, the birth process and about integrating a newborn into the existing family. As one mother said: "I can't think of a better place for sex education to happen than in the home, or a better time than when a baby is born."

The families with children present at birth seemed more likely to include the children in preparation for the baby by telling them either before the conception or when the pregnancy was confirmed about the plans to expand the family. Legg (1974) stated that informing the very young child of the anticipated birth of a sibling at least adds some reality around which the child can weave his fantasies. This group was also more likely to allow the children to participate in prenatal care by going to the doctor's or midwife's office and listening to fetal heart sounds. Children who planned to be at the birth were also more likely to attend childbirth preparation classes with their parents, and view films about childbirth.

A child's presence at birth removes the frightening mysterious implications of the mother disappearing. If the mother goes to the hospital to have a baby, the toddler may conclude that the birth was a dangerous operation (Hazell, 1969). If the child is present to observe the birth, either in the home or a birthing room, he or she can observe the well-being of the mother first-hand and experience birth as a natural process rather than a vague, frightening illness or disease.

If the child is present at the birth, there will be no unnecessary separation from the mother or father. When the mother goes to the hospital the child is likely to be anxious about the absence of the mother, worried about her condition, and resentful about her desertion of him. Many people try to minimize "separation anxiety" with gifts and promises. One obvious solution to eliminate separation anxiety is to keep all the children close by, where they can be held and talked to and reassured. Legg (1974) commented that seeing the new baby in the hospital was probably not as important as visiting the mother, especially for the child around 18 months, who may be at the height of separation anxiety.

Maintaining a continuity of presence enables the siblings to develop positive associations with the birth and the newborn. This is especially important for the youngest child, who is about to become the ex-baby. Fears of being supplanted by the newcomer make the event a potential crisis (Ward and Ward, 1976). I found that while sibling rivalry and jealousy were not completely eliminated, they were less intense as indicated by less regressive behavior of the children, less abusive behavior toward the infants and parents, and fewer behavior problems. However, in the families where the infants were at least one-year-old, at the time of the interview, there seemed to be the same amount of discord between siblings in both study populations.

RECOMMENDATIONS AND CONCLUSION

From our observations, several recommendations can be made. If children are in fact going to be present at birth, it is essential that they be prepared for this experience. In order to provide adequate prenatal preparation to facilitate a positive experience, and to anticipate concerns of the child during labor and birth, I suggest the following guidelines for the parents:

1. Tell the child as early as possible about the anticipated birth of a sibling.
2. Take the child to at least one prenatal visit with the doctor or midwife, to enable the child to meet the provider of care and to listen to the fetal heart beat.
3. Show the child colored pictures in books, slides, films, and videotapes to acquaint the child with the sights and sounds of labor and birth. Specific attention should be given to blood, which will be noticed on the mother and baby, and also to the sounds of work and/or pain emitted by the mother in the process of birthing the baby.
4. Discuss with the child the appearance of the newborn, with special attention given to the umbilical cord and the placenta. The child should realize that the cord will be cut, which will not be painful to the baby or mother. The child should know that the baby might cry, and that he or she will not be the ideal playmate immediately.
5. Try to be comfortable around the family, at least on occasion, without clothes on.

The family should obviously be the ones to determine who will be included or excluded from the birth event. Some guidelines for the family to follow with a child present at the birth include:

1. Allow the child to come and go at will, both in the birth room and the house.
2. Provide a caretaker especially for the child. This person should have no responsibility for care of the mother, should be comfortable with the child in

32

order to look after the physical needs, and should be knowledgeable about childbirth so he or she can provide answers to questions and emotional support.

3. Do not remove the child from his or her own home, if that is the site of birth, either before, during or after the birth of a sibling.

4. Wake up a young sleeping child for the birth only if there is a very familiar person who is well trusted by the child to be with the child.

5. Reassure the child after the birth that everything is all right. This should be done by both parents, but is especially important for the mother.

6. Allow the child to relate under supervision to the baby in both spontaneous and planned ways, e.g., giving a gift.

This survey led me to believe that many children of all ages have not only the ability, but the need and desire to participate as fully as possible in the birth of siblings; that many parents want to be close to all of their children, especially at such significant times as pregnancy and birth; and that health professionals will experience satisfaction by providing sensitive care to the entire family during the childbearing years.

For additional guidelines, see chapters 4 and 5.

REFERENCES

Affonso, D., "Missing pieces — a study of postpartum feelings." *Birth and the Family Journal* 4 (4): 159-163, 1978.

Hazell, L.D., *Commonsense Childbirth*. New York: G.P. Putnam's Sons, 1969.

Legg, C. et al., "Reaction of preschool children to the birth of a sibling." *Child Psychiatry and Human Development* 5 (1): 3-29, 1974.

Stengel, C., "For some birth is a family affair." *The Arizona Daily Star*. February 8, 1979, Section C, Page 1.

Ward, F. & Ward, C., *The Home Birth Book*. Washington, D.C.: Inscape Press, 1976.

3.

Birth of Siblings: Children's Perceptions and Interpretations

SANDRA VAN DAM ANDERSON

The pilot study described in Chapter 2 offers information about children at birth — through parents' eyes. Realizing that parents could possibly present a positive rationale for the decision they had already made to have or not have their children present, I wanted to explore other methods which might provide more valid answers to the following question: What role do children have at the birth of a sibling? What ideas and feelings do children have about birth? How and when do these ideas change with age, development and experience? Do children, if the opportunity is available, mature or regress through the experience of the mother's pregnancy, the birth of a sibling, and the inherent changes in the family structure? If so, how can maturity be enhanced or regression avoided by health professionals? How can readiness of siblings be assisted and facilitated? Is there such a thing as sibling bonding? If so, how can it be facilitated? Is the question of children attending birth important, and if so why?

PSYCHOLOGICAL IMPLICATIONS

The issue of children at birth might not be of such great interest if the system we now have were working well. To clarify the problems with our system, let us examine our present customs surrounding the birth of a new sibling:

1. Mother in the hospital several days.
2. Child is cared for by "other."
3. Unclear explanations to child of where mother is. This may be an effort to

34

protect him, or may be due to the inability of the child to understand verbal explanation. Child is not allowed to experience birth directly.

4. Separation handled in various ways:
   a. Talk to mother on phone.
   b. Wave to mother through hospital window.
   c. No contact whatsoever.
   d. See baby through nursery window and visit mother in lounge.
   e. Visit with mother and baby at the hospital.
5. Increased dependence by child on caretaker (father, relative, other).
6. Child may stay in another home with family friends or relatives.

ANALYSIS OF RESULTS OF CUSTOMS SURROUNDING THE BIRTH OF A SIBLING

John Bowlby (1960) studied healthy children, 15 to 30 months of age, who were separated for a prolonged period from their mothers. He observed that children go through three stages in dealing with the separation: 1) protest — fretting, crying, looking for any sign of mother; 2) despair — accepting care of the person looking after him or her, and seeming indifferent or turning away from mother when visiting; 3) detachment — acting as if mothering or human contact are unimportant.

While Bowlby's study dealt with prolonged separation, others found similar reactions to temporary separation (as a hospital stay for childbirth). However, if the child was able to maintain some relationship with the parent, the effects of separation appeared to be less harsh (Mass & Engels, 1959).

More recently, the Robertsons (1971) investigated the responses of 13 young children (17 to 29 months old) when separated from their mothers for 10 to 27 days for the birth of a new sibling. All showed behavior changes indicating emotional distress: e.g., increased sadness, lower tolerance of frustration, increased clinging and irritability. When reunited with their mothers, some showed increased hostility.

Trause (1978) collected data on 37 children at three time periods: 2 to 4 weeks before their mothers gave birth in the hospital; at discharge, when fathers and children greeted the women before going home; and one to two weeks after discharge. Data on the children's behavior was collected in questionnaires answered by the mothers, in films taken at discharge, and in naturalistic observations of both mothers and children. Seventeen mothers were visited in the hospital by their children; 20 were not visited. All children showed an increase in problems such as sleeping difficulties, temper tantrums and excessive activity. All children tended to cling to their mothers. Their mothers used more stern or angry commands at the postpartum interview.

At the time of maternal discharge there were behavior differences between those children who had visited their mothers in the hospital and those who had not. Significantly more of the non-visitors ignored, avoided and refused attention from their mothers. They also responded negatively to questions about the baby.

The author concluded, "Children do show difficulties when separated from their mothers for the birth of a second child, and children who visit show no more, and possibly less distress than those who do not," (Trause, 1978, p. 210).

Klaus (1978), in discussing the necessity for sibling visitation in hospitals, pointed out that even though there are separation problems each time the child leaves his mother after visiting her (e.g., crying, telling her to come home, worries on the mother's part), these problems are not as serious as the problems which arise if the child is deprived of all contact with his or her mother. Klaus felt there is need for more extensive visitation between children and their mothers. He, however, stops short of recommending that children be present at birth: "This is a very complex question because young children often do not react to early disturbances until sometimes months and years later." He and his colleague, Kennell, believe that a child's presence during labor or shortly after birth is probably acceptable, but the birth itself might be too confusing.

In another study of sibling visitation, Legg, et al. (1974), interviewed 21 families and concluded that those children who visited their mothers in the hospital seemed to benefit by having some of their anxieties allayed.

One might conclude, after considering the observations made on children whose mothers have left them to give birth, that there is a certain amount of emotional trauma in today's customary way of separating children from their mothers giving birth.

Since our present system of separating mothers from their families for birth causes emotional trauma, many are seeking ways to make birth and the arrival of a new baby easier on the older child. While it is true that we do not know the long-term effects on children who attend births, and that children do not perceive or understand birth as adults do, the practice may be no more traumatic than our present methods of separation. In fact, there are indications that children benefit from the experience of attending the birth of a sibling (see chapters 1 and 2).

The option proposed by Klaus of allowing a child to be present at labor but not birth may, in fact, be the most traumatic of all, because being removed before birth allows the child to see the most difficult and painful part of labor without the joyful conclusion. They wonder why they have to leave. They are left to fantasize the next step and to imagine how the baby actually comes out.

The long-term effects on children who attend births are unknown and may be worse than the effects of separation, say objectors. We do know, however, that the short-term effects of separation are much more obvious than short-term effects on children at births. At worst, the effects on children at births are subtle when the child is prepared.

When birth is managed actively with the intensive use of technology and routines it becomes more a surgical event than a physiologic one. Under those circumstances, the presence of children seems most inappropriate. In institutions, however, which have made a commitment to family-centered maternity care and which practice little or no intervention in normal births, the presence of children is one more option they can offer comfortably.

The most crucial element in successfully including children in hospital births is not a ''birth room'' or a large space, but the attitude in doctors, nurses, and parents, that birth is a normal physiologic function. Beliefs that normal birth requires delivery rooms, sterile technique, masking, anesthesia, instrumentation, and drapes, lead to practices which make the inclusion of children questionable at best. The belief that birth is a normal joyful celebration can be logically extended to the inclusion of children.

While the home setting lends itself best (most easily) to children's presence at birth, a healthy attitude on the part of a hospital staff makes it possible to adapt policies and procedures to accommodate children.

STUDY OF ATTITUDES OF CHILDREN TOWARD BIRTH

It became clear to me that if I wanted to understand how children perceive and interpret childbirth, I needed to go directly to the source and interview the children themselves. Who else would know better what they thought and felt about birth and babies than they did? Selltiz et al. (1959:236), suggests that, ''If we want to know how people feel, what they experience and what they remember, what their emotions and motives are like, and the reasons for acting as they do, why not ask them?''

Goodman (1962) and Spradley (1979) state that children are good informants, and, by virtue of their membership in society are as qualified to be informants as adults. However, they may be difficult to interview. Coles (1978) used children as informants in his investigation of the contribution of childrearing and family patterning to the development of children's perception of their world. Children's verbalizations and drawings were used to collect information. Even though Piaget used children's verbalizations as a primary data-gathering instrument for sixty years, there is an unresolved dispute among researchers about the interpretation of children's speech (Gibson, 1978). Developmental psychologists have shown that words often have different meanings for children than for adults. Some researchers suggest that early speech (that of children under the age of three years) is egocentric and reflects inability to separate self from action and from the rest of the world (Erikson, 1963; Piaget and Inhelder, 1969). Goodman (1962) proposed the use of drawings as a method of securing the child's eye view. The reluctance to verbalize often contrasts with the ease with which children respond to crayon and paper, thereby unwittingly expressing what they will not or cannot reveal in words.

Machover (1953) advocated the use of drawings with children for several reasons: it is a pleasurable form of communication; it is tension relieving; it has relatively simple instructions; and skillful performance is not a necessity. Gardner (1980:84) found that five- or six-year-old children enter a period of "passionate creativity." Their drawings begin to express their inner feelings and efforts to understand the world.

Therefore, because of the varied opinions on the reliability of interpretation of children's speech, and the acceptance of art as a vehicle of expression, I decided, in addition to interviewing the children, to use their artwork to help interpret their perceptions of birth.

DESCRIPTION OF POPULATION AND STUDY

Because of interest in the long-term aspects of the children's view of birth, their parents, and their siblings, I decided to return to the same families that I had interviewed before. Approximately one year after the initial interview with the parents, the fifty families were contacted by telephone to request an interview with the children. A total of 16 families who had home births with children present were available. Twelve of these 16 families had remained intact with both parents present; three families had experienced a divorce since the original study; and the father in one family had died. All of the 31 children in these families were willing to be interviewed and to draw pictures. Thirty of the children were Caucasian, with three of these children having one or both parents of Mexican ancestry. One adopted child in the study was black. There were 14 girls and 17 boys, who had 16 male siblings and 15 female siblings.

The comparison population included 17 families, with the parents of one of these families being separated. All of the 27 children in these families cooperated for the interview and the drawings. All of the children in this group were Caucasian, with six having one or both parents of Mexican ancestry. There were 15 girls and 12 boys, who had 16 male siblings and 11 female siblings.

Data were collected in the homes by research assistants who interviewed the children and obtained two drawings: a picture of their family and a picture of a baby being born. The children were offered a large sheet of paper for each drawing, and five different colored crayons. The children talked about the content of their drawings during and after the artistic effort. In addition, the children were interviewed. Questions focused on the child's perceptions of the birth, the parents, and the newborn; on ideas about conception; and on the child's relationship with the sibling. (See Appendix B).

RESULTS OF STUDY

The drawings and responses of children who were present at births reveal that generally the children were eager, enthusiastic, excited, and seemed to accept the experience with equanimity. Some children actively participated by doing things for their mothers, such as helping her walk, rubbing her back, or bringing cool cloths. Many of the children who seemed eager to assist were in the six- to nine-year-old age range, which corresponds with the stage of industry versus inferiority seen in six to twelve-year-old children (Erikson, 1963). The children were able to identify ways in which they helped:

I put a sheet on the bed to keep it from getting dirty from the stuff that comes out with the baby.

I gave my mother the bulb to suck out the baby's nose.

I sang Happy Birthday. (I don't remember if they brought a cake or not.)

I gave her ice chips, and helped the nurse hold things and get things.

I brought mom breakfast and brought the bucket for the uterus (ed. note: placenta).

Some children in the group not present at birth spent some time in the waiting room in the hospital. They remember such things as looking at books, watching cartoons, seeing their dad in doctor's clothes, and sleeping.

Drawings and responses of children who were present at birth reveal the children actively participating by doing things for their mothers, or waiting and watching. The three- to five-year-old children were the most likely to play a more passive role by involving themselves during labor with their own familiar toys, and then sitting quietly with a special adult to watch the birth.

DEVELOPMENT IN CHILDREN'S ART

The drawings of the children have been studied and appraised by the author and other nursing colleagues for general content and mood. It is obvious that valid appraisal of a child's drawing is not possible without taking into account the age and developmental level of the child. At about the age of two most children begin to scribble — on paper, walls, tables, sand. While two-year-olds may not start out with a plan in mind, they often will look at a scribble after they are finished and see a visual whole (Kellogg and O'Dell, 1967). When children are a little older, they will use their scribbles to make hair for people, leaves for trees, smoke for chimneys and clouds for skies. As they scribble, the movement of their hands and arms and bodies is satisfying. This joy of recording movement, known as kinesthetic drawing, gives way to the greater satisfaction of creating shapes. As children approach three years old, they show an increased tendency to make circular strokes (DiLeo, 1970). Soon children discover that the discrete circles represent a head. This is followed by the "tadpole" stage in which the human figure consists of legs coming from a disproportionately large head.

An important principle is that drawings by young children are representations and not reproductions. What is drawn is a mental impression rather than a visual observation. The children's reality is of their own mental construction; their vision is distorted by their ideas and limited by their physical capabilities. The drawings make a statement about the children themselves and less about the object drawn, as the emotional factor influences the children's concept and drawings. Thus, art is a valid representation of children's attitudes toward a subject.

Between the ages of 4 and 5 with a knowledge of the basic scribbles and shapes stored away and ready to use, children make a dramatic breakthrough. They come to the pictorial stage of their development, where their structured designs begin to look like something that adults have seen before. An enormous head at 4 to 5 is quite normal.

Piaget said that drawing consists of externalizing previously internalized mental images (DiLeo, 1973). The expression of an internal image seemed apparent in the reactions of many children. Even though the children in the study were asked to draw a picture of a baby being born, many of the children who had been present at birth drew the birth scene that they remembered, often in exact detail, including the color of the blankets and the bed springs. One child said: "This lady is wearing a green nightgown just like my mom's."

The drawings were grouped into the following categories, which were the most common themes in the drawings:

- child's eye-view of birth
- child's perception of mother giving birth
- child's perception of father at birth
- child's perception of the newborn

The following drawings have been selected for the four categories. Information provided includes the age, sex, presence or absence at birth, and selected descriptions from the children artists themselves about their drawings. The titles of the drawings and some comments have been given by the researcher. The titles represent an adult impression of the drawings, although some of them are statements of children.

CHILDREN'S-EYE VIEWS OF BIRTH

THE ANNOUNCEMENT   Girl / 8 years, 6 months / Present at birth

The child portrayed herself as the messenger. The girl is announcing: "She had a baby." The midwife is saying "Sh-h-h." A common approach used by children to create a sense of process is to draw two babies: one inside of the mother and one already born.

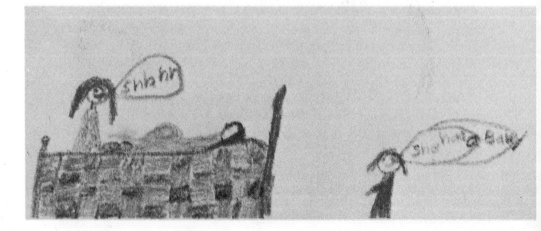

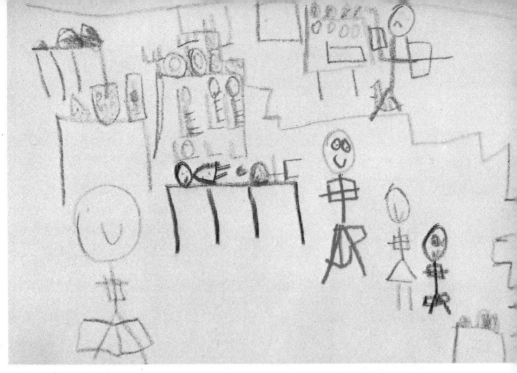

THE BIRTH SUPPER

This drawing, which includes the birth and the meal following, is full of wonderful detail. It actually contains two pictures. In the middle is Mom "with sparkles" on a bed giving birth to the baby. There are four children present — all smiling. The author had drawn himself with a brown crayon. (He is indeed black, and was adopted into the Caucasian family). The other children include one sister and two brothers. Stairs lead to the kitchen where father, with a frown, is preparing a meal, which happened one and a half hours after the birth. He has drawn plates, forks, fish, lima beans, and peas. Life goes on and the family continues with normal activity.

A HAPPY BIRTH
Boy / 7 years / Present at birth

The child described himself as "happy and jumping." The mother is "sweating and happy." "The baby is crying. There is blood on the baby. I brought my mom breakfast and brought the bucket for the uterus."

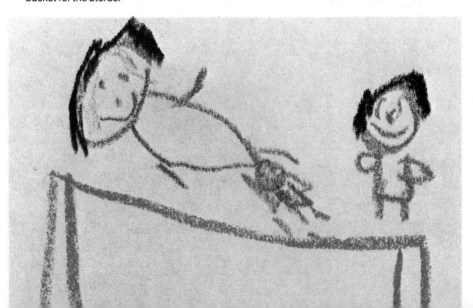

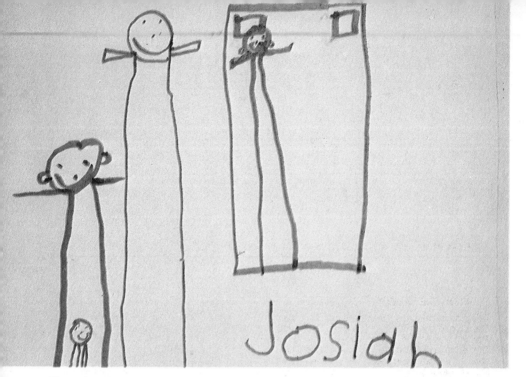

42 **PLAYMATE**   Boy / 5 years, 2 months / Present at birth

This child drew his mother in bed. Standing next to the bed is the father, and the new baby is crawling between the legs of the artist.

CHILDREN AT BIRTH   Girl / 6 years, 10 months / Present at birth

This child drew the baby coming out between the legs. The father is standing next to the mother, and the child who drew the picture, her sister, and a midwife are looking on.

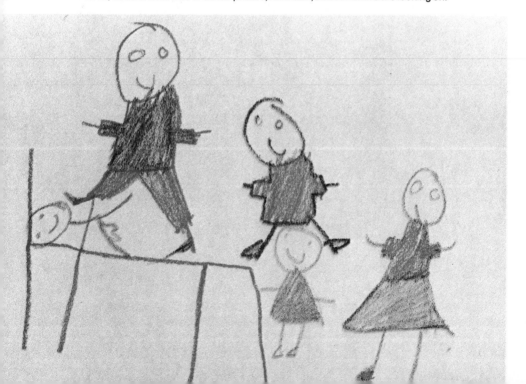

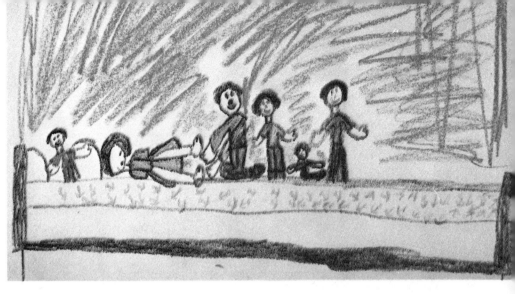

THE FLOWERED SHEETS

Girl / 8 years, 9 months / Present at birth   43

This picture displays the great detail that was often found in the drawings of eight-year-olds. The top bed sheet shows the flowered pattern that was actually on the bed at the time of birth. The child said "The bottom sheet should be flowered too, but I'm tired of drawing flowers." The father is supporting the mother with pillows. The child apologized for his small size, but he was the first figure drawn. "Mom wasn't wearing any pants. She was wearing a nightgown. Mom is getting ready to push." The other people present include the doctor, the nurse, the child and "the midwife who read me nine books." "They had to cut my mom and I ran from the room 'cause I was scared. The nurse came back and said it was all right and I saw David coming out. It was fun and I was excited and glad to be there."

BOOGER REMOVER

Girl / 6 years, 8 months / Present at birth

The picture shows the doctor at a table with the high-level technological equipment she brought: such as "things to take boogers out of the baby's nose." The elaborate black design is the headboard of the bed. Mom is in bed with baby in her "stomach," designated by the box.

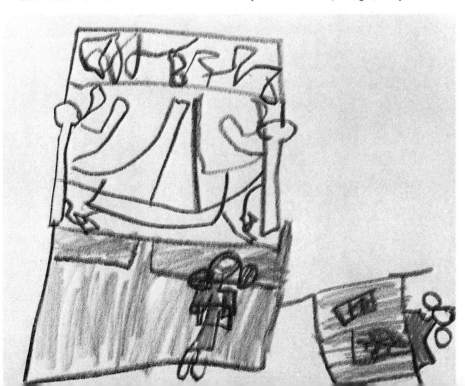

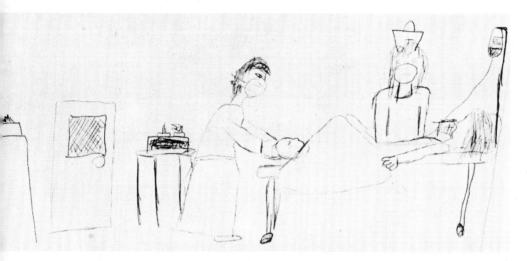

44   THE OPERATING ROOM   Boy / 10 years, 3 months / Not present at birth

"This is the operating room and here is the I.V. The lady is laying on the table. There is a doctor and nurse. The baby is about half-way out. The doctor is helping the baby out. He's about to ask the nurse for scissors so he can cut the cord. On the table is extra bottles for IV's and other supplies and there are instruments on the cabinet next tot he door."

DADDY IS HELPING   Girl / 7 years, 10 months / Not present at birth

This is the only drawing from the group of children not present at birth that includes a father in the delivery room. "The head is coming out of my mommy. My daddy is helping. My mom is lying on the bed, and is wearing a red nightgown."

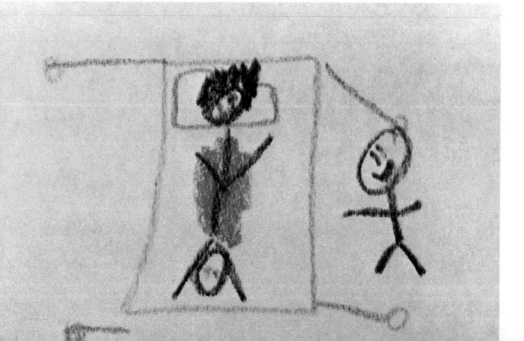

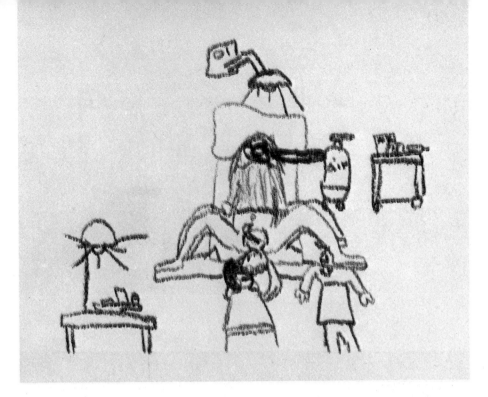

JUST IN CASE

The doctor is delivering a baby with "a lady to help" standing near him. The child drew "the things that hold her legs open," "table with syringes and things," and "air, just in case."

CUTTING THE CORD

Boy / 10 years, 5 months / Not present at birth

This child drew his mother with fuzzy hair and a blanket over. "She's not frowning, she's grunting. It's a straight face, well, if the baby's there she should be smiling. There are two doctors present, and one is about to cut the cord. There is a table with a scalpel and wrench on it." In an effort to explain the common dissatisfaction with their drawings felt by older children, this artist stated, "Let's say he is a good surgeon, but an ugly person." This comment was in reference to the large nose of the doctor in profile.

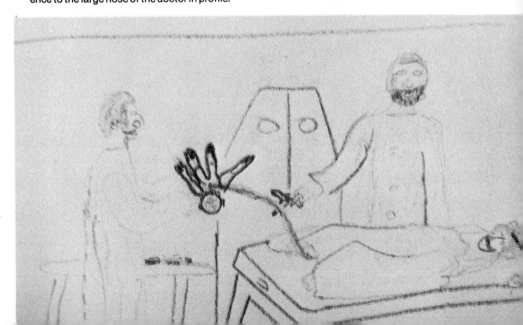

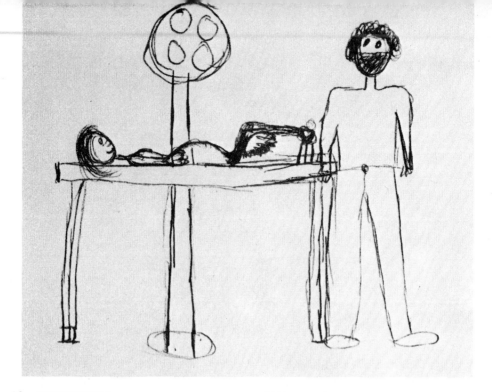

46   THE BIG LIGHT

Girl / 8 years, 7 months / Not present at birth

"The lady has her feet up in stirrups. There is a light over the table. The doctor is at the end of the table ready to help the baby."

OH MY GOD IT'S A BABY

Boy / 8 years / Present at birth

The mother and father are watching the birth of the baby.

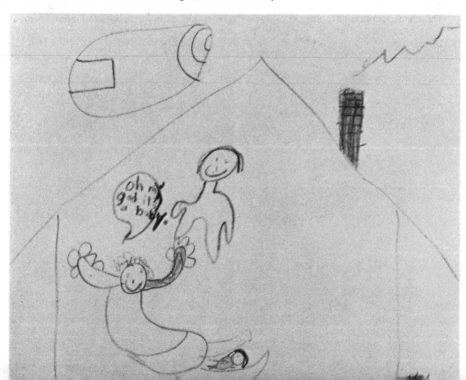

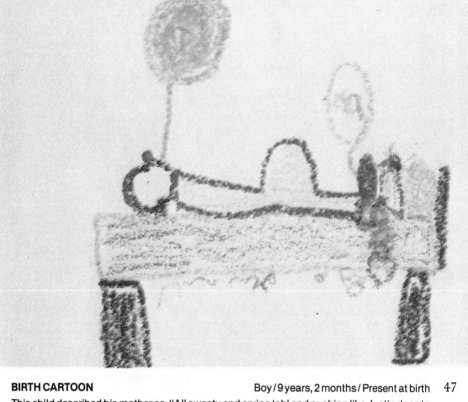

BIRTH CARTOON

This child described his mother as, "All sweaty and crying 'oh' and pushing like Justin does to poop. She is keeping her hands back 'til the baby is washed up and the cord is off." The baby's head is coming out, and the large circle had contained the word "crying," but he spelled it wrong so he colored in the lines. He carefully drew the bed springs.

WORKING HARD

Boy / 9 years, 2 months / Present at birth

The mother's face is colored blue because she is "breathing hard." "She's wearing a green nightgown just like my mom's." "The baby is being born and there is the umbilical cord." Later in the interview the child said: "I forgot to put in the blood."

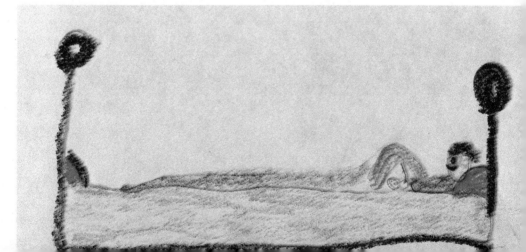

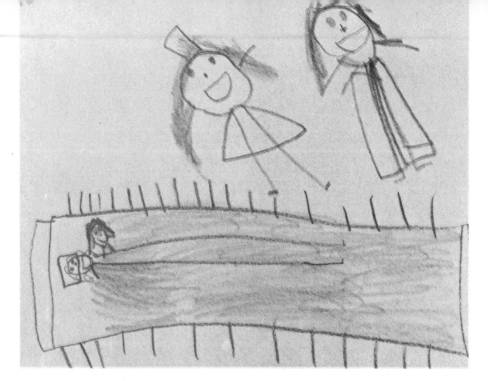

48 THE GREAT BIG BLUE COVER
Girl / 6 years / Not present at birth

"Mom is in bed with bedrails so she won't fall out. She's holding the baby, but it was first in mom's tummy. The nurse has a thing on her head and dress. The other one is the doctor."

MOM'S HEAD ON A PILLOW
Girl / 8 years, 1 month / Not present at birth

The baby's head is coming out. "That's her nightgown. Those are her legs. She's laying down not saying anything."

ALL THAT BLOOD
Girl / 7 years / Present at birth

"When the baby came out she looked like a skeleton and was all bloody. I didn't know what all the blood was about. She looked real gross but mom smiled at us and that was nice."

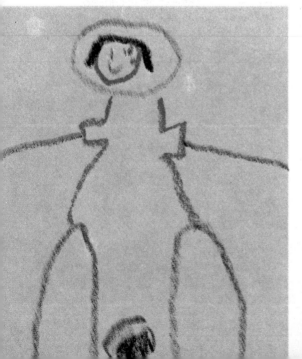

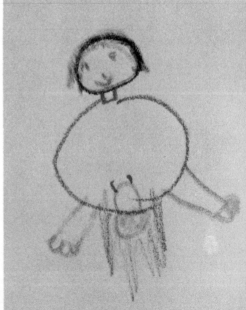

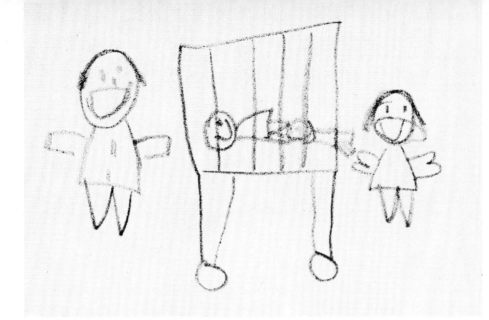

MOM IN A CRIB

"Mommy is in a crib. The baby is coming out of mommy's stomach." The doctor and nurse are wearing masks.

CHILDREN'S PERCEPTIONS OF FATHER AT BIRTH

Many of the children who were present at birth drew their fathers also present at births, either standing near the bed or sitting behind their spouses supporting them.

MY FATHER ON THE BED Boy / 5 years, 6 months / Present at birth

"My mother is on the blanket. My dad figured out she was going to have a baby and all the red stuff that came out would go on it. This is just about when the baby was about to begin. The doctor is next to the table and I'm on the chair."

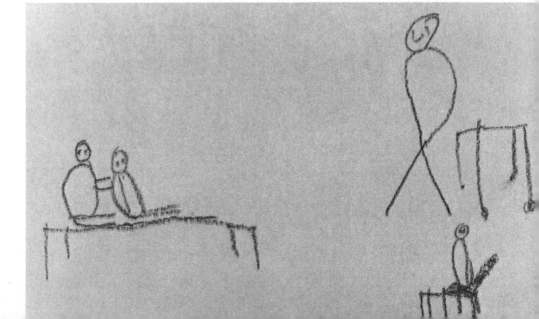

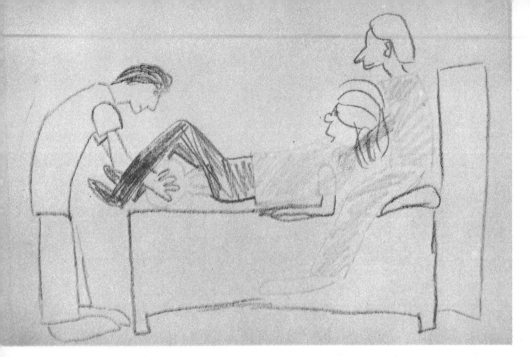

50 **DAD TALKING TO MOM**   Boy / 16 years, 9 months / Present at birth

"It was Sunday. Mom's water broke early in the morning. Dad ran around doing things. She was having contractions and then the doctor came. Dad sat behind mom and talked to her. There were mirrors at the end of the bed."

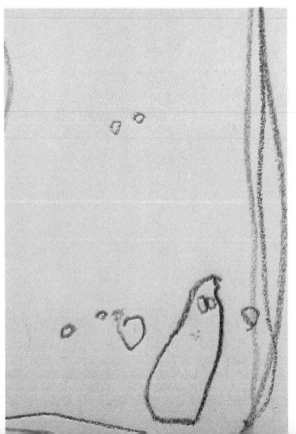

CHILDREN'S PERCEPTION OF THE NEWBORN

OUR FAMILY   Girl /
3 years, 5 months /
Present at birth

This girl drew her mother, father, and sibling in their home when we asked her to draw a picture of a baby being born.

THE WAITING ROOM

This actually includes three pictures :
1. "My dad and I are both wearing ties, and going in to see mommy. She is lying down holding Paul."
2. Mom picking up baby in her arms.
3. Sleeping in the waiting room with dad.

IN THE BOX

Girl / 10 years, 1 month / Not present at birth

"He was in a crib with glass around him. He was all wrapped. All you could see was his face. I don't want to draw the glass. His crib was next to my mom's bed. I didn't want to hold the baby because he looked too fragile."

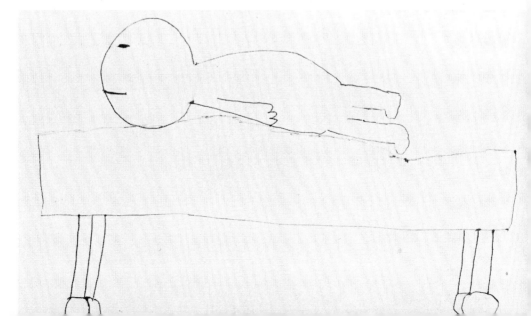

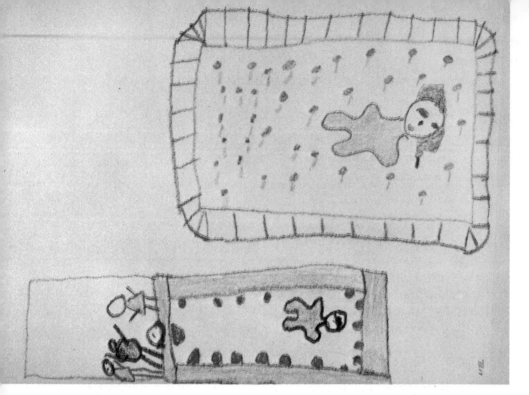

52   **THINGS WITH THE LIGHTS**   Girl / 7 years, 2 months / Not present at birth

The author of the drawing drew herself accompanied by her grandparents and an aunt visiting her new sibling through the window of the hospital nursery. The baby is surrounded by red lights ("bili light"), is wearing a black mask, and described by the child as crying. The second picture is of the baby sleeping on a blue pillow. "I put blue for his eyes but I forgot he was asleep."

The children who were present at births generally drew a family scene for the birth setting, which often included other people, usually the father and/or children. Other items which are noteworthy in several pictures are furniture, patterned sheets, smiles, and bright colors. There seems to be an atmosphere of joy and celebration. In contrast, the pictures drawn by children not present rarely included other family members. They tend to have less detail and less color. Often the woman giving birth is alone, or attended by a nurse or doctor with a mask on. In only one drawing is a father included in a picture of a baby being born. None of the drawings by children absent at births include children in their pictures. However, some of the children who were not present at the hospital births of siblings drew detailed pictures of the scene of birth in the hospital, of the doctors and nurses, and of the equipment used. Some of the equipment as described by the children, included:

— things that hold her legs open

— air just in case

— tables with IV's, syringes, and scissors

— table with scalpel and wrench

— large overhead lights

— bedrails so my mom won't fall out

— baby in nursery under lights

It is interesting that most of the technically-oriented pictures have been drawn by children who were ten years old or older and were not present at the birth. Their perceptions are probably based on books, films, television, conversations and their fantasies. They are remarkable in their accuracy. In contrast, children present at home births seemed to focus on the people present rather than on equipment.

CHILDREN'S PERCEPTIONS OF THE NEWBORN

Most of the children present at these births immediately reached out to the infant, demonstrating that they were eager to make contact with their new sibling. Some children immediately offered a special present, such as a rattle or one of their dolls or toys, to their new brother and sister. Some of the children helped wrap the infants in blankets and held their new siblings. Children were asked about their visual impressions of the babies: "What did the baby look like when it was born?" The most common response from both the home and hospital groups was something about the size of the baby. Many children commented about the hair, or lack of it.

Several children who were present at the birth were impressed by the blood and the umbilical cord. Some of their comments include the following statements:

— He had a thing on his belly. It looked like a balloon popped.

— She didn't have any hair. She looked like a little skeleton. She had an umbilical cord, small feet, small toes, her eyes were closed, her hands open, she was real soft. When she came out she looked like a skeleton and was all bloody. She looked real gross.

— He was all blue and looked gunky. His head looked big.

— I remember the top of David's head looked like a chicken bone.

These comments show that children have a rather accurate view of a newborn baby, which is very different than the usual pictures seen by most people in books of cleaned and clothed infants. The more common impression of dried, dressed babies was described by children who were not present at hospital births:

— Johnny looked wonderful, clean, wonderful and nice-looking. I'm sorry I can't put it into better words.

— He was two feet long. His arm was as wide as my thumb and he had chubby cheeks, blonde hair and blue eyes. He was wrapped up in some blankets and was sleeping.

— She looked like a little sprout (Jolly Green Giant) . . . Teeny, reddish (from the blood).

— She was pretty to me. I got to see her before my mom did.

— He was little and had a black belly button that fell off a couple of days later.

— I didn't want to hold the baby because he looked too fragile.

— Mom took us to see the baby in the nursery. He was in his box.

CONCLUSION

When the drawings in this study by children present and absent from birth are compared and contrasted, there are differences in the content and mood of the drawings. The differences indicate that children who have been included at births have a different perception of this event than children who drew pictures from their indirect knowledge and fantasy.

Because of the family scenes, the detail in the pictures, the bright colors, and the children's own descriptions of their drawing, I feel justified in saying that children who are prepared for birth are not traumatized by being present, but rather, they experience birth as a happy family event. Most of the children who were present expressed interest in seeing a baby be born. Questions about bonding between siblings needs more exploration. Based on my first two studies, I suspect that there is a special closeness in the early months which is in direct correlation to the sibling being present at the birth. However, as the years progress many other factors are involved in the dynamics of the relationship. I think this is true for all family relationships.

I believe there is no justification for excluding children from an anticipated normal birth, if the children and parents make that choice. Of course, "expecting" siblings need to be prepared for the birth event, with parents acting as major interpreteres of pregnancy, labor, birth, and newborn.

Many changes must be made in hospitals to provide the opportunity for children to attend birth if that is the choice of the family. Ways to educate children and to facilitate parental education of children must be identified. And for those families who do not want siblings to be at the actual birth, perhaps those siblings can be included in other ways both before and after the birth by being involved with the planning for a baby and in caring for a new brother or sister.

REFERENCES

Bowlby, J., "Separation Anxiety." *International Journal of Psychoanalyses* 41:89-113, 1960.

Coles, R., *Eskimos, Chicanos, Indians: Volume IV of Children in Crisis.* Atlantic: Little, Brown, 1978.

DiLeo, J. H., *Young Children and their Drawings.* New York: Brunner/Mazel Publishers, 1973.

Erikson, E., *Childhood and Society.* New York: W. W. Norton and Company, Inc., 1963.

Gardner, H., "Children's art: the age of creativity." *Psychology Today* 13(12):84-96, May 1980.

Gibson, J. T., Review of: *Eskimos, Chicanos, Indians: Volume IV of Children in Crisis* by R. Coles, in *Human Organization: Journal of the Society for Applied Anthropology* 37(3), Fall, 1978.

Goodman, M. E., "Culture and conceptualization: a study of Japanese and American children." *Ethology* 1:374-386, 1962.

Kellogg, R. and O'Dell, S., *The Psychology of Children's Art.* New York: CRM-Random House, 1967.

Klaus, M., "Future care of the parents." *Birth and the Family Journal* 5(4):246-248, Winter, 1978.

Maas, H. and Engles, R. E., *Children in Need of Parents.* New York; Columbia U.P. 1959.

Machover, K., "Human figure drawings of children." *Journal of Projective Techniques, XVII:* 85-91, March, 1953.

Piaget, J. and Inhelder, B., *The Psychology of the Child.* New York: Basic Books, 1967.

Robertson, J. and Robertson, J., "Young children in brief separation: a fresh look." *Psychoanal. Study Child* 26:264, 1971.

Selltiz, C. et al., *Research Methods in Social Relations.* New York: Holt, Rinehart and Winston, 1959.

Spradley, J. P., *The Ethnographic Interview.* New York: Holt, Rinehart and Winston, 1979.

Trause, M., "Birth in the hospital: the effect on the sibling." *Birth and the Family Journal* 5(4): 246-248, Winter, 1978.

4.

Prenatal Preparation for Children

SUSAN PARMA
and SARA PITTA
Photographs by Cindy Boucherle

As birthing practices in our culture begin to change, with the appearance of birth centers and the return of midwifery and home birth, people are wondering how to prepare siblings and other children who will attend births. In our experience, we have observed that many of the basic teaching methods which work with adults are also effective with children.

If you can communicate the essence of the birth process, and get the earthiness of it into your communications with students, they will have a good foundation, whether they are old or young. After establishing the basics, you can build with some detail, and give an idea of some of the ranges and variations of childbirth. The format, flow, length, and focus will vary with two-, ten-, and thirty-year-old students, yet the ideas you wish to transmit will be remarkably similar.

Being involved in creating a good class is akin to painting a fine painting, or producing any other work of art. It is a creative experience. It means becoming tuned in to all the participants. They provide many of the hues of which this painting is composed. Being open and sensitive to the students and allowing their energy to play a part in the direction and flow of the class is essential. Yet your responsibility to hold the brush and to give direction remains.

Of course, everyone paints different pictures; one is not necessarily better than another. We feel it's important to allow our own styles to emerge, and to nurture and develop them. If we can be open and honest with our students, the climate of the class will be more comfortable and conducive to a positive learning experience.

58

We like to keep our classes simple. There is something magical about sitting on the floor in a circle, sharing a warm cup of peppermint tea and playing with the Birth Atlas, assorted books, and birthing dolls.

HOW IT STARTED
Some of Susan's Early Experiences

Our teaching grew out of an obvious need. Late in 1976, I experienced my first birth with a child present. A five-year-old boy was an integral part of the harmonious scene into which his sister was born, after having been well prepared by his parents, and having sensitive and loving support at the time of the birth.

The second time I attended a birth with children, all did not unfold so smoothly. The difficulties were not apparent until just before the birth. In this case the birth occurred in the middle of the night. Just before the baby emerged, the father awakened his five-year-old daughter and his three-year-old son to be present for the birth. The older child, though sleepy, was obviously interested, and approached the bed where her mother was laboring. The younger child, on the other hand, pulled the blanket over his head and curled up into the mattress. The cues seemed perfectly clear, but the adults in the situation did not seem to understand them. The father began to pull at the blanket, insisting that an exciting event was about to take place, and that the child didn't want to miss it. The child pulled the blanket more tightly around him. The sibling support person sat quietly in a corner. The father insisted. The baby was born. The three-year-old dived back under the blankets, crying wildly. Fortunately, obstetrically and neonatally, events developed easily and without difficulties. For this reason, the obstetrician and I were able to turn our attention to the child and give him comfort. Shortly, the mother, being in excellent condition and being very aware of what was going on, handed her newborn babe to papa and was immediately with her three year old, holding and loving him, while he seemed to recover in her arms.

Later, as the doctor and I left the room, we both breathed a sigh of relief. His remark was, "I thought it was a bad idea to have children at birth and now I am sure of it!" My thought was, "Children who will be present at birth must be prepared. If they and the adults who will be with them are insufficiently prepared for birth, it can be very difficult for everyone. When families choose to remain together during childbirth, we must help them to prepare for the experience they are about to share." The following week, I taught my first planned sibling class.

DESIGN OF OUR CLASSES

Our teaching of children about birth begins with our first communication with the family, often early in pregnancy and usually by telephone. In this first call we attempt to get a sense of family composition, expectations, practitioner, and setting for the birth. The teaching includes actual classes with the children (usually one to three sessions), given as close to the birth as possible, as well as communications with the child and family after the birth.

ESSENTIALS
1. Understanding the basic anatomy and physiology of birth
2. Wetness of birth
3. Intensity and hard work of labor
4. Sounds of labor
5. Pain of labor
6. Episiotomy or tear and repair
7. The placenta
8. What new babies are like

We try to transmit the material from the preceding list during our first interactions. We like to follow this up by sending some material to the family which covers the same territory. The aim is to help the family talk about the birth as questions come up in day-to-day dialogue with the children. This way, when we speak about childbirth later in class, the subject is not entirely new. We see part of our role as pulling together information that has been mentioned here and there throughout the pregnancy. We also work to clarify areas of uncertainty and to give a sense of the whole of the birth process. We believe there can be value in having this learning experience happen with an adult outside the family, although we do not see this as necessary. Some families who have written to us from parts of the country where sibling classes were not available have wondered whether they could do this teaching job by themselves. Let us re-affirm at this time that while we're aware of many tools and approaches in this work that are highly effective, we believe they can be utilized in a variety of ways to good effect and can be geared to individual needs and circumstances. We strongly feel that parents are the primary and essential resource people for children whether there is an additional teacher or not.

As suggested above, under ESSENTIALS, there are a number of basic items or areas that are important to address within one's framework and through one's own style. Some teachers begin their list with conception and add basic information on postpartum and becoming a family, as well. In our work, when questions come up concerning these areas, we respond to them, or if they seem pertinent to a given family, we may bring them up. We feel this education program works well when information from the foregoing list is covered in depth, but the amount of detail we give on each topic varies with the age and development of the individuals with whom we are working.

TOOLS

Though the market has been flooded with new books on childbirth, and many are designed specifically for children, our favorite continues to be a book which, we regret, is still out of print: *Two Births*. We use it as a picture book and find it superb. We look at the photographs together, talking the children through the births. *

We draw from other books as well. A list of possible sources will be found in the appendix. We encourage teachers and parents to examine these very closely before deciding to use them. We are concerned that many books on childbirth for children are condescending, not really true to life, or too cute. We prefer to avoid these. The *Birth Atlas* and the series called "The Abdominal Cavity of a Woman," both available from the Maternity Center, are central to our teaching.

Slides and films, if selected carefully, can be very useful. We believe it's important to begin with material that demonstrates birth in its most basic form, as a natural and positive event. A new film called *Midwife,* by Michael Anderson, is a wonderful example of this. We have a vision of another film for children which shows several births, beginning with small animals and having a human birth as the final sequence.

The birthing dolls from Jan Alovus' Monkey Business have always been a favorite with the children and with us, too. For many children, it seems that handling the dolls and making the babies "get born" contributes to making the birth real. The dolls provide a wonderful opportunity for teaching and role playing about the needs and realities of the laboring woman. For example, we can play giving massage and counter-pressure to the woman, or sponging her off during active labor. We can also show the children the importance of being quiet during contractions and only communicating with the mother between them. Acting the part of mother, we can make laboring noises, including deep breathing, squeals and pushing

*Editor's Note: The book, *Mom and Dad and I Are Having a Baby!* by Maryann P. Malecki, is written specifically to prepare children to attend a birth. See Appendix D for further information.

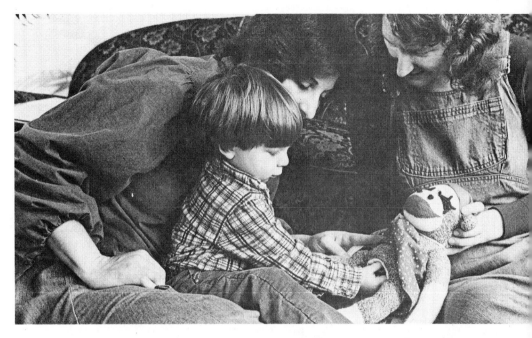

JOHN, DELIGHTED TO PLAY MIDWIFE TO BERTHA RAGS DOLL

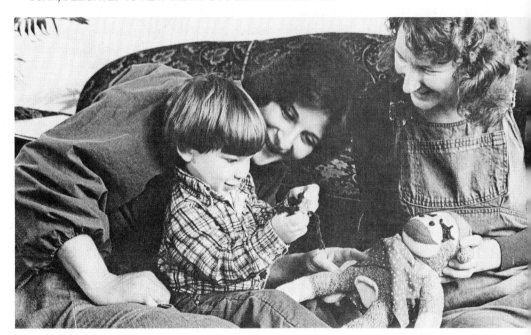

62

sounds. There is no question that the tactile experience with the dolls is powerful for the children, particularly for the young ones with limited verbal skills.

PLACENTA

Not only do we feel that the placenta is a marvelous and beautiful organ, but through the course of our teaching, we have discovered it to be an important teaching aid as well. When a three-year-old boy became upset upon seeing a placenta emerge from his mother, after having been comfortable and delighted with the birth of his brother, we decided it was time to teach children about placentas.

Since we have used a fresh placenta (in the second or third class) to teach about what it is, what it does, where it comes from, and when it is expected to arrive, not one of our students has become upset with the birth of the placenta. Though the response to the placenta is varied, from keen fascination to relative disinterest, we see that the effects of some exposure to an actual placenta before the birth itself are universally positive.

SIBLING SUPPORT PERSON

From the outset we viewed the person at the birth who was there to give the child support as invaluable to the success of the experience. In our early telephone communications with the family, we encourage them to begin to seek the right person for this role, someone who is close to the child as well as the entire family group. He or she should be comfortable with childbirth, and must not have a strong need to witness this particular birth. This person must understand clearly his/her responsibility to support the child, be sensitive to the child's specific physical and psychological needs, and be ready to respond to them as they arise. Meeting the child's needs may necessitate leaving the birthing place. There are a variety of activities that the child may need to engage in that would be disruptive to the flow of the labor and birth if done in the birth place. Taking a walk or a run and getting a meal are among these.

Within our format, having the support person attend the preparatory classes with the family is highly recommended. It is important that this person be able to explain and interpret what's going on if the child asks — verbally or non-verbally — during the experience. Being present at the classes can also help the sibling support person to feel more confident in this role.

If the birth is planned in hospital or birthing center the staff there will ideally be an integral part of the support system. Some attention should be given to familiarizing the children with the setting, as well as with the other persons who will play a part in the birth, to whatever extent that is possible. One way of facilitating this is to encourage the children to attend prenatal visits with the mother. In this way they will become familiar with the mid-wife or doctor, exams and other procedures, and also have a chance to listen to fetal heart tones.

If we are to assist the family preparing for birth, we need to have a sense of who comprises the family group, including the support person; which mid-wife or physician will be attending; and where the birth is planned to occur, be it home, hospital or birth center. This way we can tailor our classes to fit the individual family's needs.

It is important to communicate to children that they may or may not be present at the moment of birth. Since we urge mothers to ask for what they most want in labor, at each moment, we have learned that some mothers may wish for moments alone with their primary support person. This may make it necessary for the children to move out of the birth place. Complications or pure logistics can also make being present impossible for the child.

When children have a strong preference for being present but are unable to, we must be especially sensitive to them, and give them the opportunity to express their feelings. There may be feelings of disappointment or anger that need to be worked through.

Whether present or not, children, as well as adults, should have the opportunity to de-energize their experience. Paulina Perez will have more to say about this in the following chapter.

We have found it to be a more natural and successful teaching and learning experience if we work with the individual siblings or sibling groups, rather than with groups of children from more than one family. This promotes individualization and limits unnecessary distractions.

Some teachers intentionally use one or more of the developmental frameworks described by Piaget, Freud and/or Erickson when they structure their curriculum. We have discovered that this is not the way we work. While, through our own education, their work may have come to affect ours, on a conscious level we work intuitively and empirically.

Following are personal accounts written by parents whose children were present at the births of their little brothers or sisters.

STEPHANIE GETS READY TO MEET MAYA
by Phyllis Abrams

The principal reason we arranged for Stephanie (seven years) to attend Maya's birth was our view that sibling relationships are primary and on a par with parent-child relationships.

It is easy to think that children won't appreciate a situation because they can't articulate their thoughts. But in looking back, I realize that Stephanie integrated the new information about birth with a great sensitivity. Children are simply not concerned with communication in the same way that adults are. Childbirth is an extraordinary experience. To see it in all its purity is a beautiful experience for a child, far superior to romanticized protective stories.

I wouldn't have thought to seek out a birth teacher for Stephanie. But the Alternative Birth Center staff recommended one of the nurses. Sara turned out to be a practiced nurse and a wonderful, gracious lady. Her loving attitude toward Stephanie in itself positively enhanced Stephanie's feelings about the birth. Sara showed slides of births and talked to Stephanie about what to expect. The tea and cookies played some small role in Sara's charismatic image, no doubt. The sessions were a great help in establishing with Stephanie her role and giving her more specific information about childbirth.

Since Sara worked at the Alternative Birth Center, it also gave the nursing staff a chance to know us and see how we functioned as a family. It gave us a chance to know the nurses. I was especially grateful for that during labor. I felt surrounded by many loving friends.

We had made our home for the previous two years with our friends Jeanie and Totte. Totte was our cameraman. Knowing that a photographic session was going on didn't distract me in any way. We have an excellent set of pictures that we will always cherish.

We asked Jeanie to be Stephanie's support person, because she was her closest adult friend at the time. She and Stephanie are kindred spirits in that they are both graphic artists. Jeanie's room was filled with exotic objects and jewelry, artist's gear, and perhaps most fascinating of all, cloth animal friends who had lived with her when she was small.

Jeanie and Totte attended Sara's birth classes with us. This not only gave them a mental vehicle through which to relate to Stephie concerning the birth, but also served as an orientation to both the physiological process of childbirth, and the protocol and personalities of the birth center.

During the birth, in those moments when Stephanie was doubtful, I was thankful that we had had professional help in preparing her. For Stephanie, Sara was a voice of positive reinforcement in a situation that was indeed unpredictable and potentially frightening. Even though we had plenty of personal support for her, I am glad we left the teaching to the teachers.

All things considered, there isn't anything I would change about the birth.

OUR STORY OF RACHEL'S BIRTH
by Louise Rausa

Rachel sits before me, playing with her wooden, nested, Matruska dolls. She fits them into each other, exclaiming "Here's the baby!" with a child's delight each time she rediscovers the smallest doll.

Rachel's almost two and a half now, a "big girl" with huge brown eyes and a mischievous grin, and the highlight of all our lives. I'm Louise, her mother, Paul's her father, and Jeff is her eight-year-old brother. We all feel we played a special part in bringing her into the world.

Paul and I took brush-up childbirth education classes, practicing the exercises at night before we went to sleep. Jeff also took classes as part of the unique sibling preparation program offered by the Alternative Birth Center that would enable him to attend the birth. We all read a variety of books on childbirth.

The morning of Rachel's birth began like any other, but when mild irregular contractions turned into harder, regular ones, we all headed for the hospital. Upon arrival we were greeted and shown the room, which was very sunny and decorated with a rattan headboard behind a double bed, a quilt patterned bedspread, an antique writing desk, and many healthy plants. It was a friendly and secure place to have a baby.

The necessary hospital admission procedures were quickly completed while Jeff ran his little matchbox cars up and down, waiting to share them with his then anticipated little brother.

Half an hour passed and we mused over how long it would be before our baby was born. Within minutes my water broke and thick meconium, a sign of possible fetal distress, flowed with it. Chuck, our obstetrician, felt that both the baby and I should be monitored to see how the contractions were affecting the baby's well being. Because of this intervention, we were required to move down the hall to a labor room. The room didn't have the macrame wall hangings or the verdant plants of the ABC, but both my husband and son were allowed to be there. Together we waited and worked, as the fetal heart monitor clicked away, spewing forth patterns on paper telling us that our baby was all right.

I was monitored for about two hours when we were told we could return to the ABC for the actual delivery. But feeling quite comfortable and settled in to the labor room, we declined. We would move back after the baby was born.

Our baby was now ready to be born. We all had our jobs: Paul, under supervision, was to "catch" the baby, and Jeff, already our Polaroid photographer, was to cut the cord. I, of course, was to push the baby out.

A few good pushes and Rachel was out. Her cord had been wrapped around her neck and she was bluish and not crying. Paul had "caught" her, but Jeff had to forgo his job. Chuck cut the cord and quickly handed her over to two neonatologists who were standing by.

Over what seemed like a very long time, I heard nothing but the oxygen blowing, the suction apparatus going, someone calling the Lab to come for blood samples, and the words, "Dusky, very dusky . . . turn up the O_2," over and over. Then came, "Good, O.K. She's picking up. Good . . .," and she cried a loud, lusty cry. We were amazed by her size and at how bruised she was. We took turns holding her and photographing her. Then, as a preventive measure, she went to the Intensive Care Nursery for observation.

During all these events, Jeff remained close at hand. He was clearly interested in everything that was going on. He seemed completely relaxed, and to trust the hospital environment and personnel. This was scarcely a surprise to us, since he has always been familiar with the hospital setting. I have been an intensive care nursery nurse for years, and he has accompanied me to the nursery on many occasions, becoming quite familiar with medical procedures. Paul is a doctor. Amongst our friends, Jeff knows many people in the medical field. Chuck, our obstetrician, is also a long-time friend to Jeff. I'm sure this background helped him to be comfortable and unafraid through the entire experience. Jeff was interested in Rachel. He delighted in taking his turn holding her, and then he went off to see his friend.

In the end, it all turned out well. Within a few hours Rachel was given a clean bill of health from the ICN and came to stay with us for the night. She spent most of her first night sleeping on Paul's chest. The next morning we went home to begin our life together as a family of four. Jeff has always been a wonderful brother to Rachel. They've been very close since her birth, and even take turns "protecting" each other.

At this point studies are still being conducted to assess the relationship of children present at the birth of their siblings. I don't know if anything con-clusive has been documented yet, but I truly feel that it has brought all of us into a much closer family unit.

THE ZISAS SHARE THEIR STORY
by Lisa Zisa

We both came from large families. There were six children in Doug's family and four in mine. Doug had four younger brothers and sisters, and he can't recall his mother *ever* being pregnant! He missed that entirely. During his childhood there were always rivalries, especially between adjacent sib-lings. He thinks that these might have been avoided if there had been more communication between parent and child. I remember my younger brother, who came between me and the twins. When the twins came home from the hospital, he refused to walk and wanted a bottle. It was very traumatic for him. We both felt that careful preparation of our son might prevent those kinds of problems.

John is very aggressive. Aggressive, and tremendously dependent at the same time. For the first three months, he didn't sleep for more than an hour or an hour and a half at a time. During that period, he was being held, and

SHARING THE STORY OF SIERRA'S BIRTH

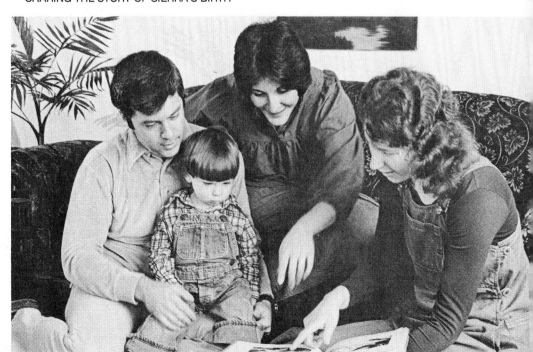

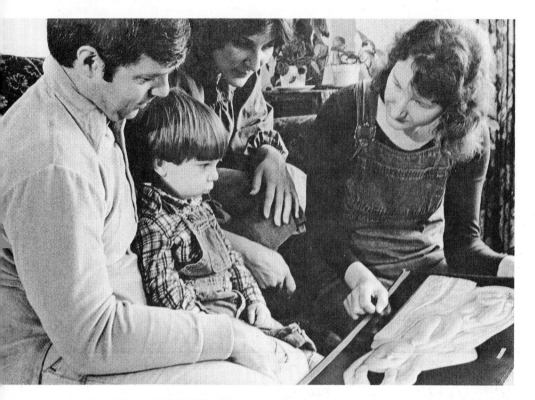

JOHN ZISA AND THE BIRTH ATLAS.

rocked, and nursed. It was so much mother, mother, mother. Since he would be only eighteen and a half months old when our second baby would arrive, we wondered how he would handle it. How could he learn to share his parents and not feel abandoned by them?

We knew right away that we needed to do some kind of preparation with John. When I was about three months pregnant, we began talking about babies to John, "Look at that baby, maybe we'll have a baby." When our midwife told us about Susan's classes, we were really excited. At first we were a little unsure as to whether John would respond to classes. We didn't know how much he would understand, at his age. When we learned that Susan had worked with children his age and even younger, we were very enthusiastic.

The classes were a benefit to John. Absolutely. Right from the start, from the first class, he really knew there was a baby in mommy's tummy.

Although during the class he didn't seem to be paying attention, later when he was running around the house, all of a sudden, he turned around and started grunting like we had done when we were pushing the baby doll out and said, "Baby, baby, baby." Then we knew it all had clicked! Of course, the graphic pictures of the fetus in utero and the photographs of a birth helped him put it all together, but we feel that Natalie, the birthing doll, was especially meaningful to him. After class we brought the doll home and kept her tucked away for a few days. When we got her out, the minute he saw the doll, he started making pushing noises and looked inside for the baby and placenta. He knew! He really knew!

We've known families where there was essentially no preparation. Maybe three or four weeks before the baby was to be born they would start talking about it. In these cases, the baby might be four or five months old before the other children really begin to realize that this baby is a person, has a personality, something to offer — a smile, for example. It might be that

THE UTERUS AS A MUSCULAR BAG

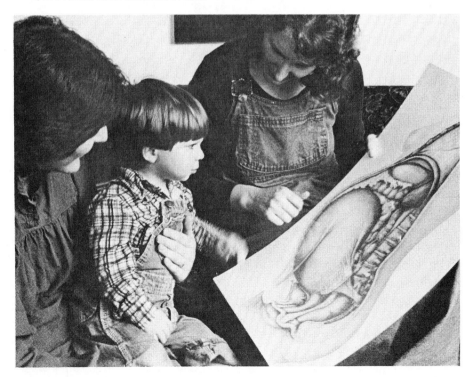

long before they would see that there could be interactions and a relationship with this baby. For the first three or four months there would be jealousy, jealousy, jealousy. We can vividly remember being at a friend's home when their little boy said, "Hey, she can smile!" But the baby had been smiling for weeks.

We chose not to have John present at the birth because of his mental and emotional development at that age. We anticipated that he would have needed us at that time; that seeing his mommy in what looks like a distressed situation he would probably want one of us to calm him. We were the only people he would have responded to, but we could not have given him any attention. We wanted to keep the birth a real positive experience. Why take a chance of having it become negative for him? If he had been a little older we wouldn't have had a doubt that he should have been there. We felt that he knew enough about the baby, that we could just bring him the next day. We also felt that it wouldn't be fair to the baby to have John present, because it would have made the baby's labor and delivery more traumatic if my mind was taken off her birthing.

In the little story book I read to John it says that the mommy's going to the hospital. Whenever I read the story to him I would whisper in his ear, "John, Mommy's going to the hospital now and have the baby." When we were leaving to go to Mt. Zion, I thought, "This is it! How am I going to do this? He's got to understand that this is it." So, while our baby-sitter held him, I went over and whispered in his ear, and he got the biggest grin on his face. He knew that this was it! He was so excited. There was never any negative reaction.

The morning after Meg was born Doug brought John to the birth room. This had been the first time I was away from John overnight and I was excited to see him, and show him his new baby sister. He ran into the room. I thought he would run into the room saying, "Mommy, Mommy," but he ran into the room saying, "Baby, baby." He just couldn't wait to see the baby! I remember my heart falling a little bit. But it was neat that he was so excited about Meg. He jumped up on the bed where she was lying and said, "Oh, baby," and kissed her, and he just really loved her already. And that at eighteen and a half months old!

After the birth, when we came home from the hospital, John was upset during the first week or so. OK, he loves this little baby, but this baby is taking his mama's time. So he experienced some jealousy. He would throw a car in her bed or try to punch her, but that began to change after that first week. Since she was two weeks old, he's never done anything to her but kiss

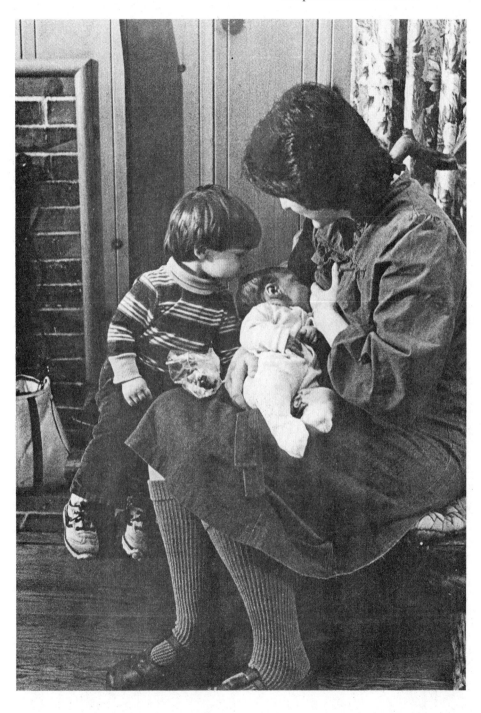

72

her or hug her. Now, if he's jealous or mad he may hit me. He will never hit
Meg. Even now, he's much more jealous of the telephone taking his
mommy's attention than he is of Meg. If I am nursing, he becomes concerned that she is satisfied. When she's done, he wants to burp her. *He* gives
her his blanket, his most cherished possession. He's always putting his
blanket in her bed. He adores her. When she cries, he calls out, "Mommy,
Mommy," very concerned. He has a real sense of her needs and a feeling
that they must be met.

As a mother, the whole time I was in labor with Meg, and going through
the delivery, I felt very calm about John and how he was, because I knew

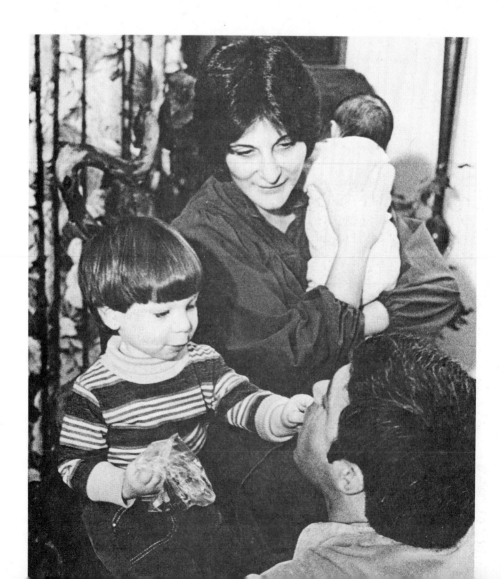

that he understood what was happening. I knew that he understood and I wasn't worried about that part. I still had fears. "How am I going to have enough love for two? Am I going to know how to take care of a little girl, if it *is* a girl (a boy would sure be easier because I've already been through that!)," but I remember having a real sense of peace, knowing that he understood. I think that made my leaving him easier. I really feel that it affected my labor and birth, because I was much calmer. Any tension causes pain, so if you are worried about children at home, or anything else, it's surely going to affect your labor; make it more difficult.

It's true that we don't know the bottom line. We don't know for sure how much his reactions stem from the classes. We've always tried to provide a loving home, a loving atmosphere for John. It's hard to say what influences in his life have caused him to be so loving to Meg. And yet, we definitely feel the preparation is still affecting what goes on here, will always affect it. Also, to have love for someone, you have to be aware of them. It's very difficult to love someone you don't know, or you don't understand.

We are glad we have exposed John to birth in such a wholesome manner.

JOHN AND HIS NEW FRIEND, NATALIE

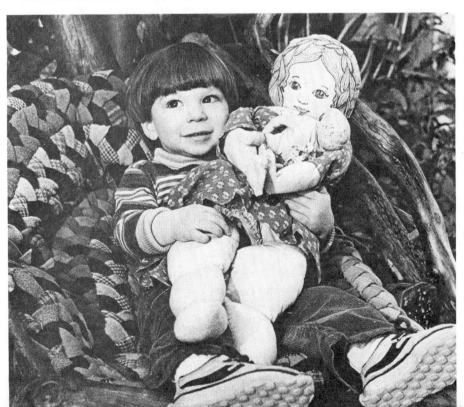

When our children are older we may take them through another series of classes. That way, Meg can be exposed in the same manner, and John can have it all reinforced.

"GUESS WHAT? I JUST HAD A BABY SISTER"
by Anne Barar

Rana's hand gripped my own. Her other hand was firmly holding Jeannine's as she watched the rapid progress of my labor. I didn't catch Jeannine's words as she leaned forward to whisper in Rana's ear, but Rana's face broke into smiles. She and Jeannine, her closest adult friend, had only weeks earlier attended special childbirth education classes to prepare Rana for the birth of our new baby and her smile confirmed that she felt at ease with the grunts that escaped my lips as I settled into the demanding contractions of transition labor. Rana, age 4, had been beside me on my labor bed since she had awakened from her afternoon nap to find me already well into labor. It seemed natural that Rana should be beside me, cuddled in Jeannine's arms, watching, not from the side lines, but from right next to me.

My waters had broken an hour earlier, signalling the onset of a violent series of contractions that had left me breathless and startled at their swift progress. Rana had slept throught the chaos of telephoning all who were to be present, through my hasty preparations for the baby's arrival and through the arrival of the midwives, my husband and Jeannine. She awoke when everyone had settled down to await the birth, and my husband Pirooz had carried her, still half asleep, into the room, explaining what was happening as he settled her gently on Jeannine's lap and she began to wake up. Her face showed neither fear nor anxiety but the anticipation of an exciting event.

"I can see black curls." Through the intensity of my contraction, I vaguely deciphered someone's words. Rana leaned across my knees to get an unobstructed view of the birth canal. I was aware of the midwife bending close and suddenly was overwhelmed with the urge to begin to push. Pirooz helped me upright among the cushions, and as I began to push the baby down the birth canal, I was only vaguely aware of Rana and Jeannine, right there with me, encouraging, assisting me. The contraction passed and as I caught my breath for the next breathtaking shove, I caught sight of Rana's hands which were holding the mirror through which I was able to watch the birth. Her hands danced with excitement. Calm voices encouraged me:

"Your baby's coming . . . reach down and feel your baby." I yelled aloud as hands gently guided mine to touch the wetness of the baby still inside me and a wave of energy flooded through me as I felt the warm, damp curls.

At this climax of my labor, I had little energy to reflect on the months of preparation that had gone into this moment. Rana had always been a crucial part of this preparation. She had visited the midwives with us at every stage, had watched our cat produce a litter of kittens and had compared human animal births in books borrowed from the library. We had made every effort to include her, to keep her informed about what was happening as the baby developed. She had helped me choose clothes for the new baby, and we had bought some extra clothes for Rana's favorite baby doll. We had also taken her with us to tour the labor and delivery suite at the hospital at which we registered in case a complication should force us to use its facilities. We felt that it was important not to shield Rana from the reality of birth, but to make sure that she was as well prepared to witness the birth of her sibling as we were. For this reason, we had arranged for her to take childbirth education classes specially for herself. At the suggestion of her teacher, we had asked her closest adult friend to share the birth and the classes with her so that she would be able to take care of Rana while Pirooz and I were absorbed. Together, Rana and Jeannine had looked at pictures, slides and photographs of births during the classes. They had acted out repeatedly the birth of Bertha's (a birthing, nursing monkey doll) baby. The reality of birth was thus not new to them.

I gave one vast shove and Darya's head slipped into view between my legs. Her first sight in this world must surely have been of Rana's face for she was right there, staring at her sister from beneath my upraised knee. I paused and pushed once more, reaching down as Darya fell into the world to take her up onto my belly. Rana followed, her face inches from that of her sister. I saw nothing but the faces of my two children, the wrinkled wet face of Darya and that of Rana, bathed in smiles as she focused all her attention on her sister. I heard my own voice crying, "I love you, I love you, Darya," and that of Rana's echoed my own. I reached to explore Darya's body and Rana slid her hand on top of mine. Together we touched and caressed Darya's skin. There were tears in both our eyes. Rana had shared with me in the most moving event of our lives and I felt the depth of the bond we had shared.

One year has passed since the birth of Darya. She and Rana enjoy an even closer relationship than I had believed possible. They act almost as I hear the mothers of twins relate, for they awaken at the same moment and fall asleep often entwined in each other's arms. Rana's love for her sister is endowed with compassion for she has experienced a glimpse of the meaning of life. She turns from play with her own friend, Tara, to consider first the feelings of sister. "Tara," she says, "let me just help Darya put her hat on her baby doll and *THEN* I can play with you."

IN CONCLUSION

It is through feedback from the families that we learn how our approach works. It is also this feedback that has stimulated us to make adaptations and to refine our education program.

Our work has reinforced our sense of the deep significance of including children in preparing for the new family member and learning about pregnancy and birth. When the child feels a part of the experience, something wonderful happens for the whole family. Birth involves a change of lifestyle for all family members. Preparation has the potential for easing this transition, whether or not the children are present at birth.

We encourage you parents to begin searching within yourselves as early in pregnancy as possible, to become aware of your deepest feelings and wishes about your coming birth. We urge you to begin early discussing these needs and desires with your practitioner. This way, in the areas where it is possible, you can claim your birth, make it your own experience. If it is your wish to have your children remain with you, and it is also what they would like, you can make plans for that possibility.

We have learned that success with incorporating children at birth depends on adequate preparation, being sensitive to children's desires and needs, and positive, nurturing support at the time of the birth.

5.

Involvement of Siblings at Birth: A Nurse's Perspective

PAULINA PEREZ

"Each child has something to teach us, a message that will help explain why we are here."
— The Talmud

The staff of the birthing center can be an integral part of the support system for the child involved in the birth process; however, many medical personnel are reluctant to work with children. Therefore, preparation of the staff of the birthing center is the first step toward facilitating the involvement of the children at birth.

PREPARATION OF THE STAFF

When parents began choosing to share birth with their children I decided to try to help these families have a positive and rewarding experience. As I worked with the families prenatally I began to realize that a supportive attitude was necessary from all the medical personnel involved. The attitude of the birth attendants was more important than the physical facilities. It was necessary for all the birth attendants to think in terms of what is important to the child and family — *not* what is important to themselves. As people became aware that I was supportive of families' plans for birth, the staff began to voice the following concerns to me:

1. I'm not comfortable with children around; they'll get in the way.

2. I don't understand why children should be involved. What is the purpose?
3. I'm afraid the children will get negative feelings about sex and birth.
4. The children will see their mother partially or totally nude.
5. The children will see their mother in pain, which may be harmful.
6. The shock of birth may be too much for children to handle.

With those who simply didn't understand why children should be involved I began by allowing them to express their concerns, comments and often negative feelings. I tried to acknowledge their feelings but also tried to help them understand that children can indeed benefit from participating in this process. Birth is truly a miracle and seeing a baby born is a unique experience. It is one of life's experiences which has many facets: hard work, pain, power, beauty and joy. When children participate in the birth process they learn to respect birth as something that requires an immense amount of effort, is sometimes painful, but which culminates in great joy. Childbirth is an experience of teamwork, and children can benefit greatly by being a part of that team. Participating in birth gives the children the same feelings as an adult who has an active, rather than a passive, role in this process. Active roles facilitate teamwork and contribute to the growth of a healthy family unit. And as one child so aptly commented when asked why she wanted to be there: "It's my baby, too."

Many people, especially those without children of their own, may be uncomfortable and insecure around children. Having a child accompany the mother to her prenatal visits gives the physician or nurse-midwife a chance to meet the child and vice versa. When a group of physicians first started working with children, one physician was somewhat anxious about a two-and-a-half year old being present for delivery, so I arranged for the child to come for a visit. The child brought his copy of *Gabriel's Very First Birthday* and "read" it to the physician. He included all the sound effects and facial expressions. When the physician realized that the child did know what was going to happen, his attitude changed and he asked the child to come back for each prenatal visit.

As the pregnancy progressed the child and physician became comfortable with each other. On one visit the child became upset and the physician asked what he was frightened of. The child responded, "I don't want you to spank my baby like the statue." In one of the examining rooms there was a statue of a doctor holding a baby up by the feet and spanking it. The physician then reassured the child that he would not spank the baby and showed him how he would hold the baby at birth. Because the child had developed a trusting relationship with the physician, he had been able to express a fear and be re-assured. This supportive attitude from the physician continued through the delivery process, which both the family and the physician enjoyed very much. This same physician is now quite comfortable with children at birth. At a recent birth he remarked to the child's support person, "This is a nice way to have a baby, isn't it?" He is truly giving sensitive care to the *entire* family. Another physician had such an impact on an eight-year-old that the child remarked: "When I grow up I'm going to be a doctor just like you."

INTEGRATING SEXUALITY INTO CLINICAL PRACTICE

It is often most helpful to hold an inservice program on integrating sexuality into clinical practice for those who will be working with children at birth. This will give the staff a non-threatening way to explore their feelings about their own sexuality as well as sex education of children. When I teach this type of workshop, new concepts and ideas are explored and the workshop ends with an exercise that gives the participants a chance to put their knowledge into practice in a clinical setting. Topics used in this exercise may include the mother who prefers to be nude in labor and the couple who use breast stimulation to enhance contractions. When people are comfortable with their own sexuality it is much easier for them to work with children's feelings in this area. If the birth attendant has negative feelings she may transfer these feelings to the child. Often nurses who have positive feelings about the sex education of their own children are the first to be willing to work with other children.

For those concerned with modesty of the human body, it is most important that they realize modesty is a family issue. This is one of the areas covered in the prenatal preparation of the family. Most families have not found this to be a problem. One mother I worked with thought she might be uncomfortable nursing her newborn with her eleven-year-old son present. We explored her feelings and she decided she would make a decision about his presence when the time came. However, at the birth this was not a problem. In fact, her son kept track of the nursing time and reminded her when to switch the baby from one breast to the other. Her comment afterward was, "It all seemed so natural at the time; I didn't give it a second thought."

Many nurses express feelings of discomfort about children being present while vaginal exams are done. It often helps if they understand that the children are aware of this procedure and its significance in labor. The children view this as a positive procedure since it has been explained that when the midwife, physician or nurse can feel a lot of the baby's head it will be time to begin to push the baby out. The gloves worn during the exam are often a source of fascination for the child and they often want to try on a pair of gloves. One six-year-old I worked with wore his pair throughout the delivery itself because he wanted "to be dressed just like the doctor."

Birth attendants may also be concerned about children watching the pushing and crowning of the infant's head. It helps for them to know that the children are aware that everyone will be looking at their mom's bottom and that the more of the baby's head you can see, the closer the birth is. If the birth attendant is enthusiastic and comments positively on the progress made during pushing, the child will usually view this with the same positive enthusiasm. The picture on page 95 shows how excited this child was when he could see the baby begin to crown even though his mother did not find pushing to be a relief sensation and was quite uncomfortable.

EXPOSURE OF CHILDREN TO PAIN

Many people express concern that if children are exposed to the pain involved in labor and birth, it will be a negative experience. Pain is something we usually try to avoid. We try to shield children from this part of the experience. Yet pain is one of life's realities. Seeing that pain can be coped with in a positive way can be a valuable learning experience for children. Perhaps if we had been exposed to this concept earlier in our lives we wouldn't be frightened of childbirth as adults. Children are taught that the pain in labor is OK. It is as much a part of the process as the hard work of pushing. Children seem to accept this pain in a matter-of-fact manner. As one six-year old commented, "It's worth it to get a baby." Birth attendants *must* have this same attitude. If they are uncomfortable seeing someone in pain they will often transfer that feeling to the child. In a recent birth, the support person for the six-year-old child became anxious during the birth. The child responded to this anxiety. At this point the nurse intervened and began to express positive comments to the child. The child then began to become positively involved with the birth again. When I saw the child again two hours following the birth, she told me about her sister's birth. She nonchalantly commented on the support person's anxiety. She was most excited about seeing the birth of her sister. She even accompanied me as I made rounds on the other patients on that floor. She told each patient about the birth. When we joined her family again she told her parents, "I made one lady's day happy telling her about Natalie being born." The nurse had been instrumental in providing this child with a satisfying experience.

BONDING

Children's participation during birth encourages bonding that occurs between the sibling and the infant. Bonding should be a family experience. For many parents this is one of the main reasons they want their children involved. Perhaps this involvement will help decrease sibling rivalry problems. The child is a part of the event and not "replaced" by the baby. With the addition of the infant the family dimensions change. Each birth is the birth of a new family. Children present at birth usually express a desire to touch and hold the infant as soon as the infant is delivered. They are often part of the massaging done with Leboyer birth. Some children have held their sibling while the five minute Apgar is done. They often express immediate concern and a desire to nurture the infant. A mother described this interaction, "I can still see Sasha, who had turned two years old on that day. I was holding Spencer and she just stroked his face all over. So gently, yet over and over. Then she had to hold and hug him." During one birth with a three-year-old present there was a delay in doing the Leboyer bath. The child remarked, "I want to take my baby home and give it a bath." He already was showing concern for his new sibling. If we were not going to give the newborn a bath he'd take her home and do it. Later he did participate in giving the infant the Leboyer bath by gently splashing water on the infant. Another family filmed their birth experience. As they viewed the film they were aware that as their three-and-a-half-year-old daughter examined her new sister she seemed to go through some of the stages Klaus and Kennell describe as steps in bonding (in *Maternal Infant Bonding, The Impact of Early Separation or Loss on Family Development*). She touched her sister gingerly at first. She then closely studied the infant's hands and compared the size of their feet. She finally patted and kissed her. Children usually assume an *en face* position with the infant. Several photographs in this chapter show this eye-to-eye contact. Some children are silent during this process but other talk to the infant as they examine it. One four-year-old made the following comments, "I know what kind of hair he is gonna have — RED! He doesn't say any words. He has little tiny ears — it would be funny if a baby had big ears. Oh, he put his finger in his mouth." After this exploration time the same child introduced his new brother to everyone. He said to his brother, "This is Daddy — his name is Steve. This is Mommy — her name is Mary. This is Granny — her name is Waldron. I'm Bradley."

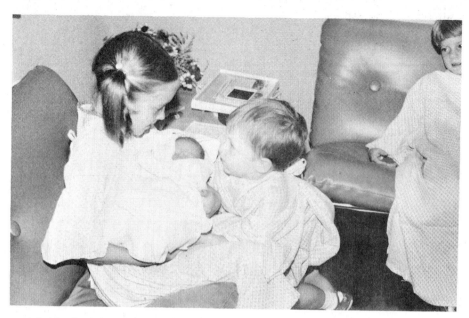

Julie introduces Lauri to her baby brother.

Sheri and Lauri one-half hour after birth.

Sheri couldn't resist kissing Lauri.

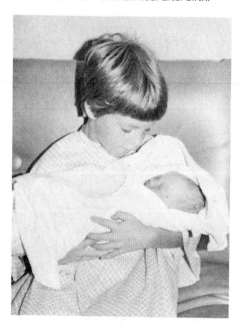

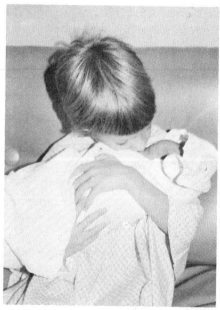

For those families who choose not to have their children present at birth I *strongly encourage* them to have their children come into the birth area as soon as possible after the actual delivery. I feel that the children will feel less of a sense of loss of love from their parents if they are allowed to participate in the birth in some way. This bonding time is important for all children. As one mother explains, ''Jessica was very serious when she held Spencer for the first time. Now she has a deep love for her brother and I know it was starting then.''

Rusty inspects Lauri's feet (after inked footprints were done) while the rest of the family poses for pictures.

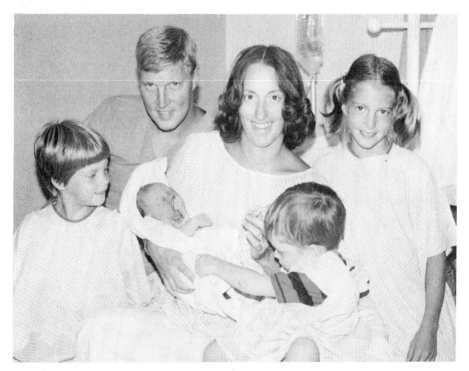

CONTACT BETWEEN EDUCATOR AND STAFF

It is often most helpful for those doing the education of the children prenatally to meet with the staff of the birthing center. This can be done with an informal meeting or a scheduled inservice education program. The teacher

84

can explain to the staff the material she covered with the children as well as the feedback she gets from them. It is important that the staff knows that the child has been emotionally and intellectually prepared for the birth. This meeting also gives the staff an opportunity to view any dolls, books, films, or videotapes used in the children's preparation. I would strongly encourage the educator working in a new area to attend several births of families she has worked with so that the staff can *see* the positive interaction between the child and a health professional. The staff can see first hand that not only do the children benefit from the experience but that the birth attendants benefit also. I also share the families' positive comments with the staff after the birth. I leave copies of the children's essays and letters as well as the parents' evaluations of their experience with the staff. They are usually put on a bulletin board in the coffee room. This way all personnel receive feedback about the couple's experience.

After the medical personnel have been exposed to this information they are usually less reluctant about working with children. As staff members work with children, their attitudes often change for the same reason mine did. It was the children who made a believer out of me. It gave me a new perspective when I began to see birth through children's eyes.

Julie adopts the *en face* position.

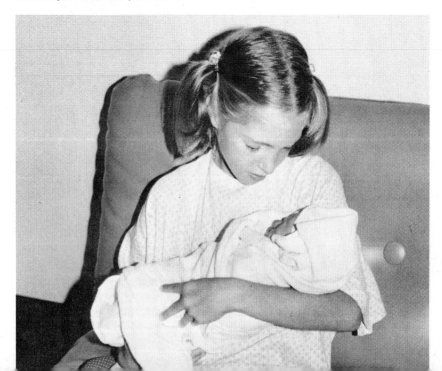

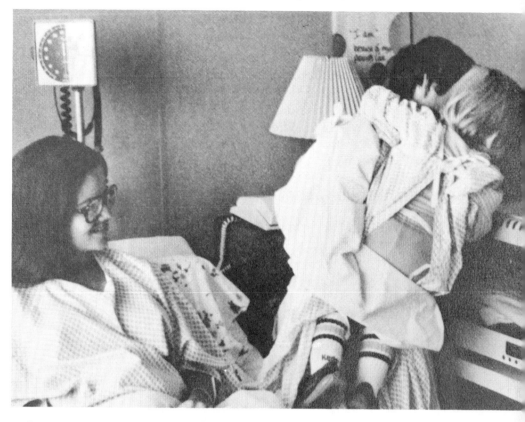

Daniel wants to be sure Adam is OK in there.

Daniel and dad watch as Adam breastfeeds for the first time.

Daniel, almost two, holds his new brother while his mother, grandmother watch.

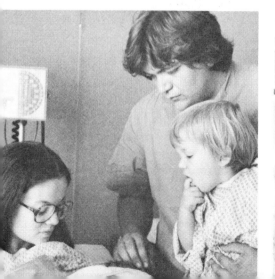

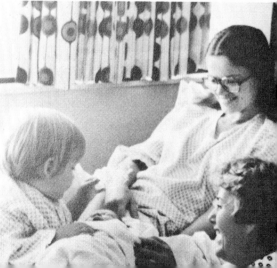

ORIENTATION OF CHILDREN TO THE BIRTH CENTER

The staff's first contact with the child may be at the orientation to the birthing center. Part of the orientation should be directed toward the child. The support person for the child should come to the orientation also. A supportive person who is sensitive to the child's needs is instrumental in facilitating an active satisfying role for the child. This person may be a close friend or relative. A grandmother is often the child's support person. Grandmothers are likely to be very excited about witnessing a birth as many were heavily sedated for their own children's births.

The trip to the hospital for the orientation may be the child's first visit to a hospital. As the nurse talks with the parents it is often helpful to have a scrap-

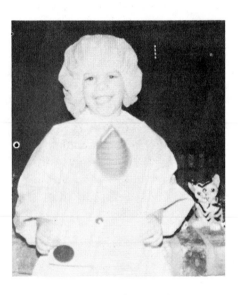

Amy with her big sister certificate after her sibling tour at Woman's Hospital of Texas, Houston.

book of birth photographs available for the child to look through. The child's part of the orientation could begin with the nurse discussing the photographs with the child. She can assess the knowledge base of the child by asking pertinent questions about the photographs. I prefer for the photographs to be in color and graphic in nature so that they are as close to the real experience as possible. Labor and birth can be reviewed in this manner, and the role the child wants to play in the birth process can be ascertained. It is most helpful if notations about the child can be made on the mother's hospital records, as these records are usually readily available to the nurse in attendance during labor.

Children are often fascinated with the placenta. If possible, it can be helpful to have a placenta available at the orientation so that the child can examine it. If the orientation is done in the birthing area the nurse can show the mother the birthing bed by allowing her to "try it out." When the mother assumes the position she would like to be in for birth, a role play of the birth can be done. I often ask the mothers to emphasize and dramatize the sounds of birth so that these will not be frightening to the child at the actual birth. If the orientation is done in an area other than the birthing room it is helpful to have a birthing doll or monkey doll available to role play with.

At the Woman's Hospital of Texas in Houston the children have a hospital tour all their own, as well as participating in the birthing room orientation. This sibling tour includes a tour of labor and delivery, making fetal monitor strips of their own heartbeat, making fingerprints like their mothers will do for the birth certificate and learning how to hold, diaper and feed an infant. The tour ends with each child receiving the disposable cap, gown, mask and shoe covers he/she wore on the tour as well as a diaper to use for practice on a doll or stuffed-toy, a big brother/big sister certificate and a tee shirt that says "Certified Big Brother" or "Big Sister" on it. The children often wear the tee shirt to the birthing room orientation and/or the birth itself. After the tour one three-year-old asked her mom, "Are you going to have our baby here?" When the mom said she was, the three-year-old said "Oh, good!" The director of nurses also sends a congratulatory letter after the birth to each child who participated in the tour. This hospital also has a "sibling touch program" which involves a birthday party for the family. This program allows the child limited access to his/her mother and sibling between 6:30 and 9:00 P.M. in the evening.

When the nurse meets the family being admitted to the birthing area she should make a special effort to familiarize the child with the environment if this has not been done before. The child is often fascinated with the equipment used in the birthing room — the fetoscope, doptone, and sphygmomanometer. As she demonstrates these, the nurse explains how they will be used in labor. The child may be familiar with these, if he/she has accompanied the mother to her prenatal visits. The child is usually free to feel or touch anything in the room. However, if there are certain things he/she should not touch, the rules about these should be explained.

NURSE'S ROLE IN LABOR WITH A CHILD PRESENT

When the mother is in early labor the nurse can spend time with the child since the parents need less help from her. She begins to assess the knowledge base of each child. Questions which may be helpful include:

1. What is mom going to do while she's in labor?
2. Did you see any movies about babies being born? What was your favorite part of the movie?
3. Does it hurt to have a baby?
4. Which part of the baby will we see first?
5. What will mom sound like when she's in labor?
6. What will mom sould like when she's pushing?
7. Do you want to be here when the baby is born?
8. What do you want to do during the labor?
9. What do you want to do after the baby is born?

Answers to these questions help the nurse determine what the child wants out of this experience. She also often learns why this particular child wants to be involved. When one child was asked why she wanted to be there she simply stated, "It's my baby too." Others may make comments about specific things they want to do. They often express a desire to be the first one to tell if the infant is a boy or girl. They often want to touch and/or hold the infant immediately after the birth, to help with the Leboyer bath, or to be the first person to diaper the infant.

If children bring books about birth, the nurse can use these to explore their knowledge of and feelings about birth. The nurse may ask the children to show her some favorite photographs. She may look at the photographs with the child and ask "What is happening in this picture?" The answers to these questions will vary with the age, personality and concerns of the child. Children often bring their birthing doll or monkey with them. Asking pertinent questions and by having the doll give birth with appropriate sounds, the nurse is able to assess the child's knowledge. As this assessment is being done, the nurse should take into account the age and level of development of the child. She will also observe the child's interaction with his/her parents, other siblings, support person and any other people in the area. She makes an effort to introduce the child to all personnel who enter the room.

As labor progresses, the nurse should explain all procedures. She may remind the child about things learned prenatally, as they apply to labor. For instance, it is a good idea for especially young children to be reminded that contractions are the mom's uterus squeezing hard against the baby and that these contractions tell the baby to come out. She should remind the child to be very quiet during a contraction so that mom can concentrate on her relaxation and breathing. Reminders about the birth process should be used throughout the labor. One six-year-old arrived at the birth center while his mother was in transition. The mother was being most vocal about her displeasure with this part of labor. The child asked, "Is that my mom yelling?" I answered that it was and the child's response was, "She yells like that at home sometimes, too." We spent a few minutes talking about this part being the hardest part of labor but the child did not seem to be disturbed by his mother's discomfort.

Even in a flexible birthing area, labor may be boring to a child. As one older child told me later, "The movies I saw didn't show the boring parts." If it is night the child may bring a sleeping bag so that he/she may sleep awhile. It may also be helpful to bring books, games, toys, and cards for amusement. If it is not a distraction to the mother, the child could bring a record to play, as many birthing rooms have a phonograph available. Some birthing areas also have a television. If snacks and juice for the sibling are not readily available at the hospital, these too can be brought from home. The child should also feel free to leave the birthing area with the support person at any time.

The nurse can comment on the events of labor and offer suggestions on how the child can be an active participant. She may discuss the topic of pain as it is happening. She acknowledges that the mother is in pain, reminds the child the mother is OK, and offers ways to help the mother. For example, the nurse might comment, "Mom's not smiling right now. Her contractions are hurting her a little and she's having a hard time relaxing. Maybe you could get her a cool cloth for her forehead and remind her to relax. Maybe we could ask her if she wants ice chips." If the mother is walking during labor the child can walk along with her. Older children may even help with breathing techniques. An almost-three-year-old explained transition by saying, "Then Momma said HELP." When asked what happened next he replied, "They helped her."

Some families choose for the children to stay at the home of the support person until the active phase of labor. When one six-year-old arrived at the hospital after spending part of the day with his support person he brought his mother a bouquet of flowers he had picked. His comments when he entered made it clear to all present that he had a good knowledge of what happens in labor. On the trip to the hospital he had spilled some of the water from the flowers on his pants. When he entered he remarked, "I'm all wet. I feel just like a pregnant woman when her water breaks.'' Families who choose for the children to arrive during the active phase of labor should be aware that sometimes labor progresses rapidly. If this happens the child may miss the birth. This has happened to several of the couples I have worked with.

As vaginal exams are done, the nurse can remind the child that she is trying to feel the baby's head and that when she feels a lot of it the mom can begin to push the baby out. When pushing begins she can comment to the child that pushing is very hard work. I often tell the child that pushing the baby out is a little like climbing a mountain. It is very hard while you're doing it but you are very happy when you've finished it. Birth is often not quiet. The child has been taught about the noises of childbirth but I often find it helpful to remind the child of the film he/she saw. I also comment that the mom is OK and that her body is made so that it can stretch as she pushes. Often, between pushes the mother will comment to the child about what's happening. One mother said, ''The baby's head is making my bottom burn but that's a sign it will be born soon.'' Another commented, ''Mom is hurting now but I'm OK and the baby will be born soon.'' When one mother was pushing and making noises her three-year-old asked, ''Is mom crying?'' She was reminded that those were pushing noises. As the baby began to crown she excitedly announced, ''Oh, it's a BABY!'' If oil is being used for perineal massage this should be explained to the child, I usually explain that the oil helps the mom's bottom to stretch more so the baby's head can come out. The same six-year-old who brought his mother flowers in labor stood at the end of the bed as his mother began to push. The physician then let him sit on his lap at the foot of the bed and his eyes began to sparkle as he could see the head when she pushed. When he could see the head he told her, ''Push harder, Mom. I can see the baby! I can see the baby!'' One three-year-old girl had a very similar response as she coached her mom to ''Push hard, push hard, it's almost here.'' Some children have commented that as the head begins to crown it looks ''funny and weird.'' One child said, ''It doesn't look much like a baby's head to me. It's all wrinkled.''

During the pushing the nurses usually fill the Leboyer bath if this is to be used. Often older children may want to fill it themselves. The nurse can assist younger children.

If an episiotomy is needed for the birth, an explanation of this should be given to the child. The nurse may choose to direct the child's attention away from the episiotomy as it is done. One six-year-old girl viewed the episiotomy very positively as she commented, ''It was easier to push the baby out when the doctor made the cut.''

During the delivery itself the physician, the nurse, or the child's support person may "talk the child through the birth". The nurse should allow the child to relate to the birth in any way he/she chooses. Some children are very verbal and involved. In one birth such a child told the physician he was "wasting those gloves by using them just once". Another commented, "I can't see — the doctor is in the way." Other children are very quiet and somewhat awe struck. As one mother explained, "It wasn't what she said at the birth but how she looked." The nurse or doctor often makes comments such as, "Mom is blowing so the baby's head comes out slowly," or "It's hard work to push the baby's head out." When the baby's head is delivered the children are most excited. One three-year-old who badly wanted a baby sister exclaimed, "It's my baby Holly!" when only the head was born. When one baby opened his eyes before the body was born his brother said, "He's looking at me. I think he likes me." Children sometimes narrate the delivery of the baby's body. A child's comments were, "Oh, look the head — now the shoulders and . . . it's a GIRL!" One six-year-old was so excited after the birth of his sister that he ran out of the birthing area to tell the other family members waiting outside. As he left he asked his mom, "Can't they come in and see her?" The mother agreed and the extended family came in to share his joy. A pictorial essay of this experience is included later in this chapter.

The umbilical cord is often a point of fascination for the children. I remind, especially the younger children, that the cutting of the umbilical cord is not painful to the baby. As one four-year-old boy explained to others later, "It didn't hurt when Daddy cut Blake's cord. This was the cord that was hooked onto Blakey." A three-year-old said after the clamping and cutting of the cord, "Her belly button sure is bigger than mine now. When she gets bigger hers will look like mine." Some children ask to feel the cord and are allowed to do so.

As the placenta is delivered the nurse can remind the child that the blood involved is OK and natural. I sometimes tell the children that the blood is the food the baby doesn't need any more. Physicians have been quite helpful by stopping and showing the placenta and membranes to the children. The picture on page 98 shows the physician making this explanation. Several older children have asked to put on gloves and examine the placenta and were allowed to do so. One eleven-year-old said before the delivery that she did not want to see the placenta. However, she became so involved with the delivery process that after the delivery of the placenta she asked us to "show me both sides of the placenta." Some of the children aren't that impressed with the placenta though and tell me "it's weird."

AFTER THE BIRTH

Children often ask to be the first to hold the baby after the cord is cut. Some children have held their new sibling while the five-minute Apgar is done. Other children may want to wait until the baby is "cleaned up and not yucky." As one three-and-a-half-year-old girl explained, "When Jessica first came out she smelled as bad as a walking stick (an insect that smells bad)." The children seem to begin to develop an attachment to their siblings during this holding and bonding process. It can be quite awe-inspiring to watch this sibling closeness with the infant so soon after delivery. The children are often very protective of the newborn. One three-year-old girl questioned us when her new sister was placed in the incubator. She asked, "Why are you putting my baby in a cage?" Another six-year-old child held his new brother for the first two hours. When the nurse needed to do the hourly assessment on the infant he questioned, "Do you have to bother my baby again? He's sleeping." One of the personnel marveled at a six-year-old sitting still for two hours and offered to hold the infant so the child could get up and move around. The child refused the offer, saying, "No thanks. Kyle likes it here."

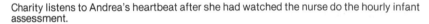

Charity listens to Andrea's heartbeat after she had watched the nurse do the hourly infant assessment.

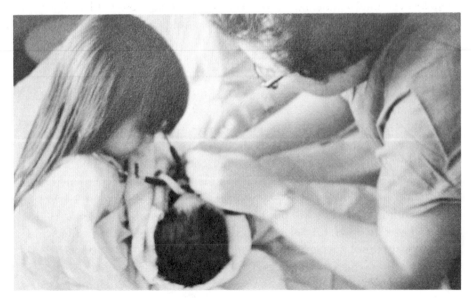

It is most important for the nurse to explain to the children all procedures and exams done with the newborn. At one birth the nurse did not explain the need for the vitamin K injection and simply gave the injection. When the infant cried the six-year-old brother was most concerned and big tears appeared in his eyes too. We immediately stopped and explained the need for this injection and also discussed the booster immunizations he had to receive before starting school. After this he seemed reassured and was not tearful or upset. This type of interaction was avoided in another birth when the nurse took the time to explain to the four-year-old brother why blood tests on the baby were necessary and how the infant would react. The brother was not upset when the infant began to cry and consoled his new sibling by saying, "It's OK. I'll hold you in a minute and you'll feel better." Pediatricians have been supportive by explaining the newborn exam to the sibling as well as the parents.

Families often have a birthday party or celebration of some kind in the immediate postpartum period. Gifts from the sibling to the newborn and from the newborn to the sibling are often exchanged. The sibling often views the newborn as a gift to the family. A good present for the new baby from the sibling is a record of uterine sounds. This will be useful during the postpartum period in the hospital as well as at home. Some children want to pick this gift themselves and a special shopping trip has been devoted to this purpose. One three-year-old chose a small teddy bear for his new sibling and when he presented it to the infant he explained, "Here is your teddy. I have a big teddy." When he put the bear in the bed with the infant he remarked, "Oh, he likes it." This birthday celebration often includes juice for the children, champagne for the adults and birthday cake for everyone. The siblings often celebrate the infant's birth again with their peers at school by passing out cupcakes, suckers or bubblegum cigars. As one father explained, "I'd never before seen Clay get up and want to go to school early, but the day after Emily's birth that's exactly what happened. He couldn't wait to hand out suckers and tell about Emily's birth."

It is critical that the events of the day be discussed with the children after the delivery. This can be done by the parents, birth attendants, or the birth educator. It is important to *listen* to the children and get a sense of what they thought and felt about the delivery. Often all questions after the delivery are directed to the parents. Everyone asks, "How did it go? How did you feel? What did you do?" The children should still be made to feel like important participants in the birth process. Ask them to "talk about your baby's birth." When the children are talking it will be helpful for you to consider the following questions. These questions will help you to ascertain how the children have integrated their experience into their lives. You will find that children absorb what they are ready to accept.

1. Is the child's story spontaneous?
2. Are there are parts of the experience that were confusing to the child?
3. Does the child feel good about herself/himself?
4. Is the child happy with the ''new'' family unit?
5. Is the child happy about the experience?
6. Is the child happy about the new baby?
7. What was the child's favorite part of the birth process?
8. What did the child not like about the experience?
9. Was there anything scary?

It is during this time that any misconceptions or fears come out. If something unexpected or frightening has occurred, there must be a way for the

Tad alternates playing with toys and watching his new brother Jason.

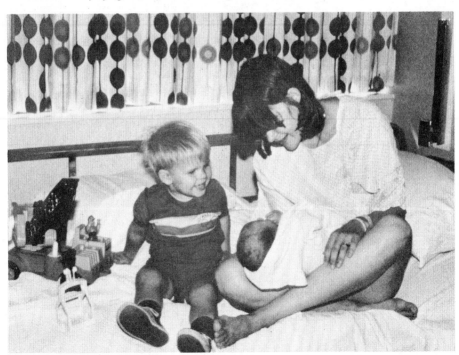

child to deal with it as soon as possible. Avoid having the child feel a sense of helplessness. Information and explanations can be given. The child can be held physically close and reassured. Children seem to incorporate this birth experience into their lives rather quickly. After the birth they often alternate between playing with their toys and showing interest in the newborn. The picture on page 94 illustrates this. A nonchalant attitude after the birth is often the sign of the child's natural acceptance of the birth process. Children do not seem to have the need to verbalize as much about the experience as the mother and father do in order to integrate this experience into their lives.

BENEFITS TO ATTENDANTS

The birth experience is gratifying for the attendants as well as the family. Helping children participate in the birth of a sibling can be a powerful and moving experience. Working with children has changed my life as well as theirs. Watching a child's eyes dance and sparkle as she sees the baby emerging from her mother's body has been most rewarding. One mother explained this moment perfectly by saying, "I'll never forget the look on Clare's face as she saw the baby born. It was one of the most thrilling experiences of my life." What compares with hearing a child welcome his sibling into the world? Before the infant's body was even delivered one child had welcomed his brother with, "Hi, baby!" The newborn opened his eyes and the sibling's excited comment was "Look, I think he likes me!"

Adults can learn a great deal about life by working with children when life begins. Children can add such joy to our lives — sometimes with a simple comment. After the birth of her sister one three-year-old approached her mother, gently patted her on the cheek and softly said, "Thank you, Mom." What can replace the feeling you get while watching a child hold and rock his new sister fifteen minutes after her birth? One three-year-old sat and sang songs to his new brother. Watching a children begin to attach and form a bond with their new siblings is most touching. But the feeling is much stronger when you begin to realize what an impact these moments may have on their relationship. Eleven months after his brother's birth one seven-year-old child commented: "Sometimes when he gets into my toys and messes them up he drives me crazy but I just love him so much." Moments such as these are the reasons I am enthusiastic about working with children and their families. Sharing births with children has helped me to truly appreciate the miracle of birth. Seeing birth through a child's eyes has helped me to see the wonder and beauty of life.

Following are stories by children who were present at the births of their siblings. All photos were by Paulina Perez, except those on page 104, taken by Fred Catrett, and on pages 96-99, taken by Kathy Sudela-Proctor.

NICOLE'S BIRTH
by: Christy Carlson — age 11

When my mother first told me she was pregnant it was hard to believe. I was very surprised. After my mother had been pregnant for a few months, I got used to the idea that I was not going to be the only child anymore.

When my mother came into my room one night, and announced that she had to go to the hospital because she had started labor, my heart jumped!

After 16 hours my mother was finally having the baby. When I first saw my little sister she was like a dream. I thought it was wonderful!

Now whenever I hold my little sister I think about my experience in the birthing room. You know, I don't think I would love my sister like I do if I hadn't seen her being born.

BABY EMILY'S BIRTHDAY
by: Clay Williams — age 6

Clay's eyes sparkle as the baby's head is born. His birth educator "talks him through the delivery."

Clay coaches his Mom to "push harder;" while he sits on the physician's knee.

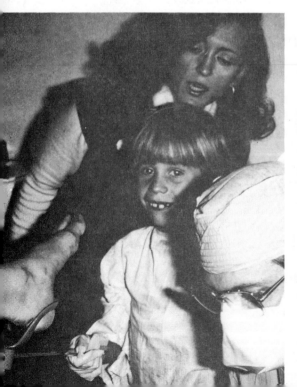
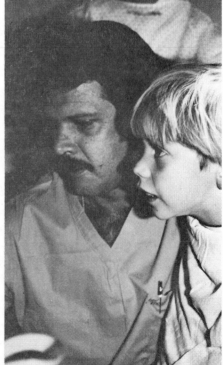

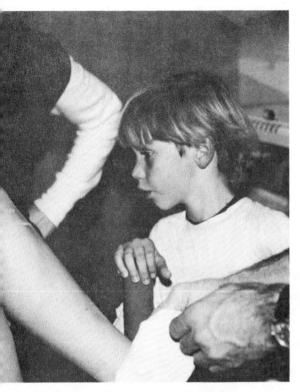

Clay wanted to watch the delivery from the end of the bed.

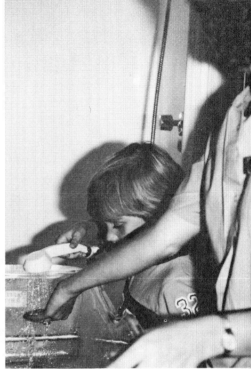

Clay fills the Leboyer bath.

When I woke up I was so exicted and I said, "What?" I thought Mom was waking me up to go to school. But when she told me she was going to the hospital I jumped out of bed and got dressed in a flash. Then we got into the car and drove to Kathy's house — my Mom and Dad drove to the hospital.

At Kathy's house, she baked breakfast, while I got dressed in my regular clothes. We ate breakfast and went to the park. When we got back from the park, we fixed some flowers for my Mom. I watched cartoons for awhile, then we went back to the park. Then we got the call to come to the hospital.

*I went to the hospital. I put on a gown and washed my hands. The baby was starting to come out and John, the doctor, was wasting too much gloves. I said, "John you're wasting those things!" And he said, "That's okay. Your Dad's going to pay the bills!" I saw the baby's head coming out and I said, "Okay, Mom, **push!**" And John said when he saw the baby's shoulders, "What is this, a man or a baby?"*

98

Then the baby was born and I felt so happy. I went out into the hall and invited Grandma and my aunts to come in and see my new baby sister. My Grandma and my Dad were crying. Pretty soon my Gramps came too.

I went to get a coke. Aunt Susan cut the cake and served champagne.

The nurses from the nursery came in and so did her doctor. The doctor checked her heart and the nurse gave her a shot. Everybody wanted to hold the baby and I was the last one.

Then we went to Mom's signed room and Dad and I went too. I finally got to hold the baby. Then Dad and I went home. I couldn't wait to go to school the next day and pass out lollipops to all my friends!

The "new" family immediately after the birth of Emily.

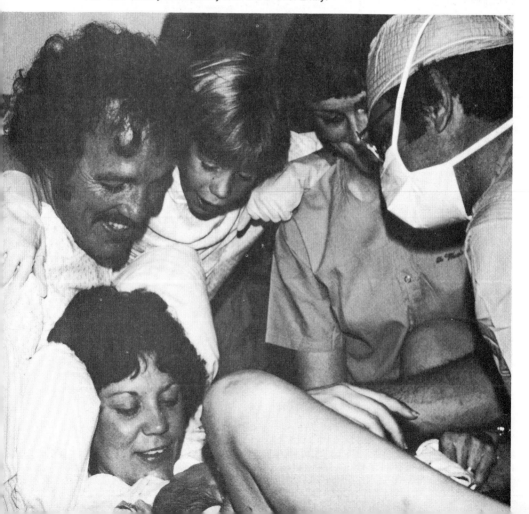

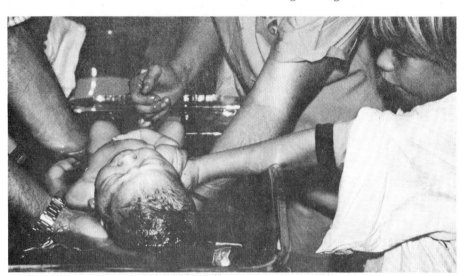

Clay enjoyed helping to hold 10 lb. 2½ oz. Emily for the bath.

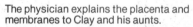

The physician explains the placenta and
membranes to Clay and his aunts.

Clay nuzzles with Emily as his dad calls
friends to tell of the birth.

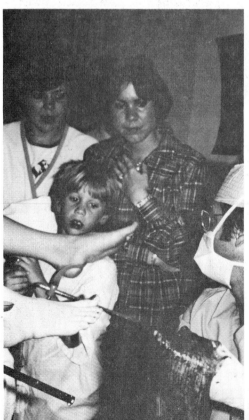

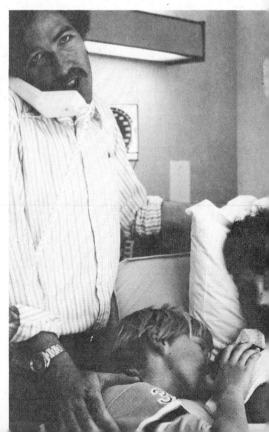

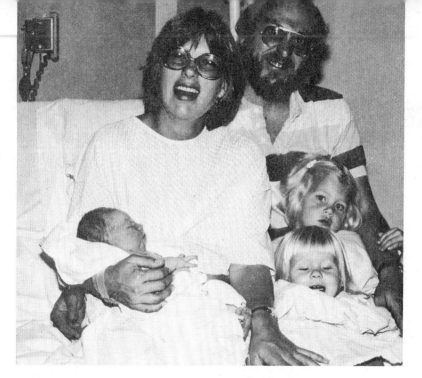

The first "new family" portrait — Vicki, John, Spencer, Jessica and Sasha.

JESSICA, SASHA AND SPENCER
by: Jessica Nolley — age 3½
Sasha Nolley — age 2

When Spencer was born we went to meet him. He was eating. We touched him. Then the nurse made us put on yellow paper gowns. We touched him some more. We patted him and hugged him. Then we sat on the bed with Mom and took his blanket off and looked at all his parts. We liked the warming bed. We had our pictures taken with Mom, Dad and Spencer. Then we had a party!

Jessica holds Spencer while Sasha impatiently waits her turn.

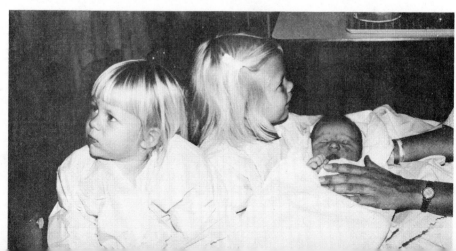

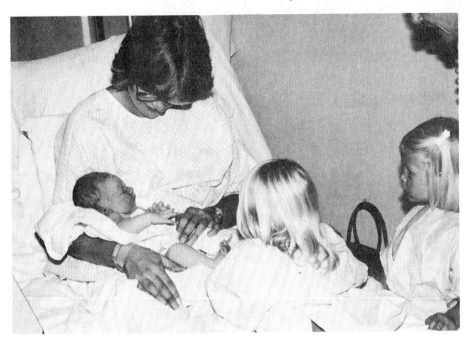

Sasha and Jessica examine their 10 lb. 14½ oz. brother.

WENDY BIGGS'
BIRTHING ROOM EXPERIENCE

by: Wendy Biggs — age 6

When I got to the hospital I was so excited. I thought it was going to be a boy. When we got to the birthing room my Daddy got me some ice chips. When my momma done her contractions I felt sorry for her. When I saw the orange stuff that they put on my Mamma I sure didn't like it. I don't know why they put it on her. When I saw the baby's head it had the prettiest hair. And then Dr. Leeds came in and then I put on my gown. And then Dr. Leeds cut Momma and it scared me a little. And then the baby slipped out and it was a girl and we named her Natalie. I got to hold the baby and she was so sweet. And I hugged her and I kissed her. And then Granny came and got me. I was so glad I got to be there to see my little sister be born. It really was a lot of fun.

MY SISTER'S BIRTH

by: Ryan C. Wolfe — age 2¾

Daddy and Mommy woke me up real late. I went to Grandma's. I waited for Daddy to call me so I could go help Mommy borned baby Holly. I went to sleep on the floor at Grandma's by the telephone.

Daddy called and me and Grandma runned to Grandpa's truck. Grandma went real fast. We got to the hospital and took a ticket. We went way up and left Grandpa's truck.

Mommy was walking around and around. I helped Mommy blow.

Dr. Leeds told Mommy to push. She made a face and some noise. Mommy said, "Help." I was next to Mommy and I pushed hard too!

I saw baby Holly's head first. Then her body was borned. She was all messy and needed a bath.

The nurse put a binky (blanket) on my baby and I holded her. Baby Holly needed a bath. Grandma holded her.

I was hungry. Me and Grandma ate pancakes and bacon. Me and Grandma went home to play and wait for Mommy and Daddy to bring our baby home.

Mommy and Daddy came home soon (8 hours later). I ate chicken and holded baby Holly. She was clean and asleep. She was pretty now. I went to bed. I was tired.

Ryan as he took his "Baby Holly" home.

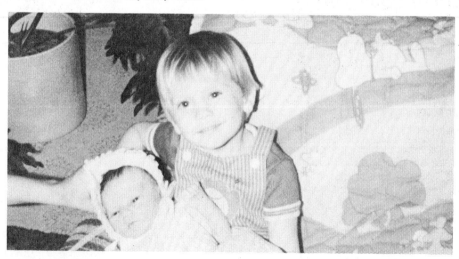

THE BIRTH OF KYLE DAVID   by: Troy Coleman — age 10

My dad woke me up at 3:30 am. I decided to go to the hospital and miss a day of school. I had perfect attendance and hated to miss a day of school but I wanted to see the baby born more than going to school. I felt tired. Chad and I went to a friend's house and went to sleep. We woke up at 7:30 am. We ate breakfast and a friend took us to the hospital. While we were driving she was excited a lot. I was excited, too. We got caught in the rush hour and she thought we were going to miss the birth of the baby. We saw my mother before she had the baby. We only saw her for abut five minutes. Then we had to go out of the room. Then we came in and the head was barely out. My mother was in pain. Dr. Leeds, our doctor, kept asking me, ''What do you think, Troy?'' I didn't know what I thought; it was just neat. Then the glorious moment happened! The baby was born! It was a boy and we called him Kyle David. We got to hold him and diaper him. I liked it a lot. I didn't like it when he was in the nursery and I couldn't hold him.

Chad was the first person to put a diaper on Kyle.

The hourly newborn exam is done while Chad holds his brother.

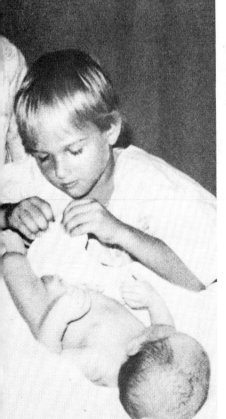

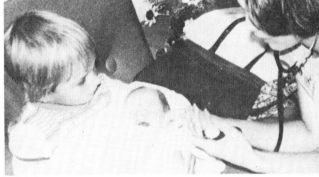

Troy holds Kyle while younger brother Chad watches.

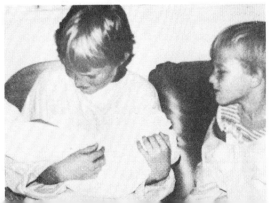

"MAMA PUSHED OUT BABY JESSICA OUT OF HER UTERUS"

by: Marie Catrett
— age 3½

I went to see the hospital. I got a certificate saying I'm going to be a big sister, and we wore a little mask like a doctor wears.

Well, Mama came and woked me up, and she said, "Marie, it's time for Jessica to be born." So she waked me up, and I said "Oh boy! Mama! I'm so glad." Then Mama and Daddy took me over to P.J.'s house, and I slept with them, and then Nonnie and Sampa came and picked me up. You know what she did? She just kept her arm around me. Well, we went up to the hospital, and so I heard her cry, and I said, "That's my baby! Let's go get her! And so I holded her, and Nonnie and Sampa came up with me.

She was kinda pink, and wet, and she had a little cord on her. She smelled bad as a walking stick (an insect that smells bad when touched). Well, I ate myself's breakfast and then I ate my Mama's breakfast, and I ate all of Jessica's birthday cake too!

I helped Mama and Nonnie get Jessica dressed. I put her hat on her, and then we brought her home from the hospital. I wanted my baby to sleep in my room, but Mama said she might get hungry in the night, so we put her in Mama and Daddy's room. When she gets bigger she can sleep with me.

I'm glad we could go to a special hospital where I could get to hold my baby. The big brother on **Sesame Street** *didn't get to hold his baby. Next time I think I'm just about old enough to help Mama breathe, and I bet I'll be the first one to see the baby.*

Big sister Marie holds Jessica.

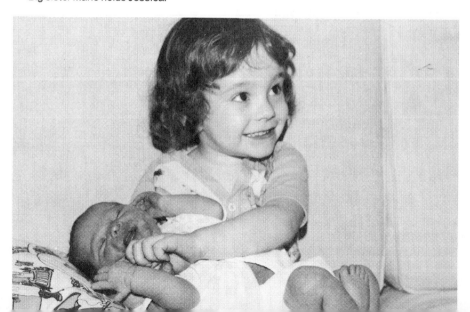

BRADLEY'S STORY   by: Bradley Godken — age 4

You were pushing, and Blake came out. It didn't hurt when Daddy cut his cord. This is the cord that was hooked on to Blakey!

I saw Blake in his incubator. He used to be a seed. Now he's my brother.

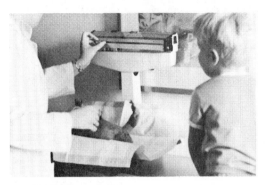
Bradley watches the nurse weigh Blake.

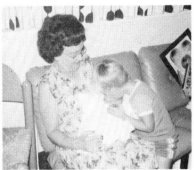
Bradley kisses his new brother while Granny watches.

THE DAY MY BABY GOT OUT   by: Jeff Ireland — age 5

My Mom had been growing a baby for a long time. I couldn't sit on her lap anymore. We read books about babies. My baby was like a fish in a bubble inside my Mom. I wanted a sister.

I came home from school and my Mema said my Mom and Dad had gone to the hospital to get my baby out and I had to take a bath and eat my supper and put on my dress clothes. Mema and I went to the hospital and I knew where to wait. After awhile my Dad came in a doctor's suit and said, ''Come see your new brother!''

I was so excited. When I got in the room I hugged my Mom. She said to go over to the box to see my baby brother. He was so little and he wiggled a lot. My doctor was looking at David so I sat on my Mom's bed until he finished. A nurse got me a coke.

I got to hold my baby and he liked it. I love my baby so much. I can teach him a lot of things because I'm five years old and very big.

My Dad and I went and got hamburgers because Mom said she was starving to death. I got to hold David again.

I helped my Dad bring Mom and David home the next morning. I am so happy my Mom had a baby.

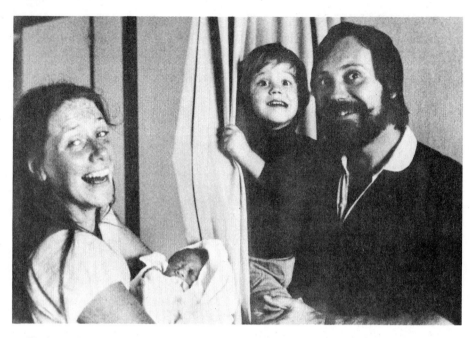

The happy Vellucci family — Ron, Helen, Danny and Joey.

Scott and Shane admire Shane's new sister.

Danny gently strokes baby Joey.

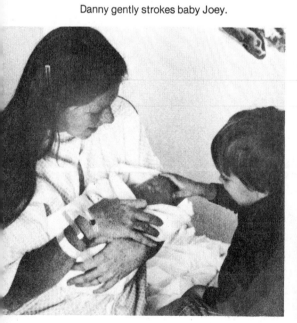

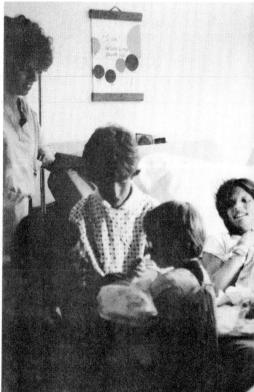

WHEN BABY JOEY
WAS READY TO POP OUT

by: Daniel Vellucci — age 3

One night when I was asleep, Baby Joey got ready to pop out of Mommy's belly. Mommy and Daddy woke me up and Daddy carried me outside to the truck all wrapped up in Ba (my blanket). I wanted to go to the hospital but we had to go to Laura's house. It was too late and I had to sleep. I cried, but Laura hugged me. I was lonely at first, but that was because Mommy and Daddy weren't there with me.

When I woke up I wasn't lonely anymore. Laura made a special breakfast for Josie and me; it was pancakes, my favorite! Then Laura and I went to the hospital. We were going to meet Baby Joey. But first we stopped and brought him a present — it was his birthday!

When I first saw Baby Joey I liked him pretty nice. He looked like me! He was still kind of dirty from the greasy stuff and bloody, though. But we didn't give him a bath yet. Mommy showed me his umbilical cord, the incubator bed and the bottle of sugar water.

Later on, Josie, Laura, Dick and I all had a birthday party with Mommy and Daddy for Baby Joey in the birth room. We had champagne and birthday cake.

It was pretty nice.

Baby Joey came home with us that night. He likes to drink a lot of milk. He is still very little but I like him and kiss him and sometimes I can hold him.

SCOTT'S BIRTH STORY

by: Scott Perez — age 8

Since my Mom goes with kids who see babies born, I asked her if I could go with her to see a real live baby born. One of the Moms named Anne said I could come when her baby was born. Four months later I asked when was I ever going to get to see that baby born? Well, that night my Mom woke me up at two in the morning and told me now was the time for the baby to be born. So I dressed in a hurry and we went to the hospital. The baby's brother, Shane, was there and he and I played together until it was time for the baby to be born. All of a sudden there was a lot of hurrying and they told us to wash our hands and put on gowns. We stood right behind the Dr. and watched the baby be born. It was a girl. Shane and I helped his Dad give the baby a bath. After the baby ate we both got to hold her. Then I had to go home and go to school. My favorite part of that night was all of it.

Birth is for Babies, Children and Loving Beings
*(Who See the Wonder and Beauty in Life)**

*By Cheryl Wines and Gloria Gould in *Children at Birth,* Marjie and Jay Hathaway, Academy Publications, Sherman Oaks, CA., 1978.

6.

Cesarean Birth Through Children's Eyes

ANN ARMSTRONG SCARBORO
and PENNY SIMKIN

INTRODUCTION

Today in the United States between 10 and 20 percent or more of all births are cesarean sections. The number varies from community to community, depending on the ages and circumstance of the women giving birth and the kind of health care practices existing in the community. It is generally true, however, that the number of cesarean births is increasing and an ever-increasing proportion of these cesareans are for women having repeat cesareans. The number of childbirth preparation classes designed specifically for women who will have cesarean sections is also growing.

This trend toward a greater number of cesarean births has coincided with a general practice of including children more directly in the events of family life, including birth. As a result, parents are seeking accurate descriptions of cesarean birth to share with their children. Parents having cesarean births want to help their children feel a part of the birth although they may not want them to be present for the operation itself. They need to know how children perceive cesarean birth in order to give an appropriate explanation.

In recent years many prospective parents have come to feel that birth should involve the father as well as the mother. The proliferation of childbirth education classes which emphasize the father's role in supporting the mother during the birth has affected cesarean births too. Fathers who have attended classes want to be part of the birth experience even when the birth becomes a surgical procedure. Mothers who have anticipated sharing the birth want the fathers' support even more when the birth becomes complicated in this way.

The first cesarean birth in a family is almost always unexpected and unplanned. While recognized as difficult for mother and father, this can also be very difficult for the children, especially if they have been looking forward to being present at the birth but then the need for surgery prohibits their attendance. The nurses and the parents will need new language to describe a cesarean birth, and the children will need extra support because their parents may experience emotional trauma about the birth.

From the perspective of the family, a cesarean birth means that hospitalization, anesthesia and surgery are absolutely necessary. It means that the mother will be away from the family longer than she would be for a vaginal birth, and it means that her recovery will be at least slightly longer and different. She will not have as much energy for meeting the needs of the children, they won't be able to sit on her lap, and she will have to be allowed to rest and recuperate from the operation.

If it is a repeat cesarean section, the parents can take time to explain everything to the children ahead of time. The children can plan to share the event by being present in the hospital and ready to meet the new baby just as soon as possible. Hospital support personnel can plan to be with the children during the surgery and be ready to help them meet the baby.

HOW TO DESCRIBE CESAREAN BIRTH TO CHILDREN

Two books by the noted psychologist, David Elkind, *A Sympathetic Understanding of the Child: Birth to Sixteen,* and *Child Development and Education — A Piagetian Perspective,* are particularly helpful in finding the best way to explain cesarean birth to children. Elkind points out that we should use the correct terms immediately in conveying information to children. He suggests that what an individual experiences in the way of feelings and emotions depends both upon the circumstances and on his level of development.

Parents and health care providers should give simple, precise explanations of why and how cesarean births occur. One could say, for example, "In a cesarean birth, the doctor makes a small cut called an incision in the mother's abdomen. He/she makes another incision in the mother's uterus. Then the doctor lifts the baby out of the uterus and through the incision and the baby, cord, and placenta, are born. Then the incisions are sewn up. The mother receives medication before the surgery begins so that she does not feel the incisions."

Children who are planning to attend a birth, either in or outside the hospital, need to be prepared for the possibility of an unexpected cesarean, or transfer out of the home, birth center, or birthing room. Stories of births where a cesarean became necessary, told in a simple and matter-of-fact manner, can help prepare children for this possibility. The role of the children and their feelings should be included in the story. The children should then have a chance to ask questions and explore their own feelings, as well as what they should do in the situation.

As an example, the following story might be told (with modifications suitable to the sex, age, interest, and situation of the child):

THE SMITHS' BIRTH STORY

The Smiths were all so happy when their new baby was coming. They were going to have their baby at home. Dr. Sam Jones was coming to help with the birth and so was his nurse, Mary Johnson. The Smiths' big boy, Scott, was 6, and he was going to be with his mom and dad when the baby was born. Scott's grandma was coming from California, too! They made a birthday cake for the new baby.

Then the big day came! Mom went into labor, Scott took a bath and put on clean clothes and played all morning. Mary Johnson came, and so did Dr. Jones. Scott played all afternoon, wandering in and out of his mom's room to see if the baby was coming yet. It sure seemed slow. Mom came out and played a game with Scott, and took a shower and had something to eat. She was getting real tired of the labor. After supper, Dad told Scott that Mom's uterus had slowed down and wasn't working real well; that's why it was taking so long. He said he and Mom and Dr. Jones and Mary thought they'd better go in to the hospital to get some medicine to help Mom's uterus. Dad said Grandma and Scott could come too, but they'd have to wait outside Mom's room. Or they could stay home and Dad would call as soon as the baby was born. Scott was getting kind of sleepy, but he wanted to see the baby born. Dad told him that the rule in the hospital was: no children until after the baby is born. Scott cried. He was all mixed up. Grandma came in and said, "Why don't we stay here together and we'll drive straight to the hospital as soon as the baby is born, even if it's in the middle of the night. Your Mom needs some help in the hospital because labor isn't working quite right." So Scott watched while everyone but Grandma went to the hospital. Mom said she was sorry, but she needed the hospital. Scott went to bed, feeling kind of sad.

The next morning Dad called and told Scott he had a baby sister who was very big for a baby. She was so big she couldn't fit through Mom's vagina, even when they gave the medicine to help her uterus. So at 6:30, just about when Scott was getting up, they decided Dr. Jones should do a cesarean. A cesarean is when the doctor cuts open the mom's skin on her tummy and her uterus, and takes the baby out through the opening. Then he sews the opening back up. The mom can't feel it because she has medicine to take away all the feeling. She gets a scar on her tummy.

At 7:30 the cesarean was done. Dad told Scott to come quickly to the hospital with Grandma to see Shelby, his new sister. Scott and Grandma raced to get ready. Then they got the birthday cake, and went to see Mom and Dad and Shelby. Mom was kind of sleepy. She just smiled and said, "Hi, Scott. This is Shelby. She's a fine sister for you." Everyone ate some cake and sang "Happy Birthday" to Shelby.

A discussion following the story might include questions on why Scott cried, how he probably felt, why they did the cesarean, why the hospital doesn't allow children, etc.

Parents should be encouraged to debrief the child afterwards, explain their own disappointment and explore the child's feelings.

The reason the mother has had a cesarean (or will have, in the case of a planned cesarean) should be clearly and accurately explained. For example, "The baby is too large to go through the mother's vagina or pelvic girdle;" "The baby is supposed to be born head first and this baby has its buttocks coming first;" "The baby is lying crossways so that the head cannot be born first as it should be;" "The cord is wrapped around the baby so that it will get pinched and the baby won't get enough oxygen during the birth;" "The mother's previous baby was cesarean and there is a chance the uterus might rupture."

The explanations must be geared to the age of the child. Children of two or three years old will most likely not ask questions, but they will probably hear the term 'cesarean section' at some point during their mothers' pregnancies or immediately afterward. A brief explanation is one way of including them in the event. Elkind adds that children need recognition, and that answering their questions is a way of rewarding their symbolic expressions of themselves. If the answers are clear and brief, the children will be satisfied without being confused.

Human beings learn in different ways. Some people learn best by hearing, others by doing or by seeing, or by various combinations of these methods. Visual aids enhance learning, and the illustration on the following page is offered for this purpose. Another visual aid which parents might find useful is Natalie, the birthing rag doll, or Bertha, the birthing monkey doll. Natalie's address is given in Appendix C. She can give birth by cesarean section as well as vaginally.

There is a brief but accurate account of cesarean birth in *Inside Mom* by Sylvia Caveney. A new book, *Special Delivery, A Book for Kids about Cesarean and Vaginal Birth* by Baker and Montey covers the subject very well (see Appendix D). It is difficult to find books on the subject. Of the 22 books in the Phoenix public library on the subject of birth for young people, only 5 even mention cesarean birth.

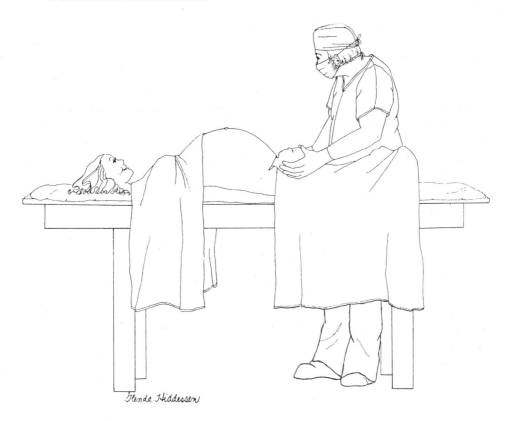

Glenda Hiddessen

Books about children and operations may be helpful in preparing children for the birth of a younger sibling. Examples are *Jeff's Hospital Book* by Harriett Langsam Sobol, *Curious George Takes A Job* by Hans Augusto Rey and *We Are Having a Baby* by Viki Holland. None of these involves a cesarean birth, but the first two do include hospitalizations and the third is about birth.

Children, like adults, tend to personalize experiences about which they hear. If the child who is learning about cesarean birth is a girl, it would be wise to emphasize the fact that her babies will probably be born vaginally, because she may assume that her births will be like her mother's.

THE IMPORTANCE OF PARENTAL ATTITUDES

Elkind also points out that young children are sensitive to adult moods and feelings. The general literature about parents and cesarean birth is full of examples of frustration and disappointment. Richard Hausknecht and Joan Rattner Heilman, in *Having a Cesarean Baby,* say, "Women whose cesarean births have been difficult times for them can carry the emotional scars around for years, especially if they bottle up their feelings within themselves and then feel more guilt because they have them."

Bonnie Donovan, in *The Cesarean Birth Experience,* quotes a mother who said "I do not understand the operation. Three months later I still wake up with nightmares." The mother of a two-and-a-half-year-old girl who was born by cesarean section said that she could not really relate to the child, that she didn't like her much, and that it had something to do with her birth. The nurse who told this story said that the father does the nurturing in that family.

If parents are upset by their cesarean birth experience, they need to explore their feelings and try to resolve them before they begin to discuss such a birth with their children. Otherwise, their negative feelings will color the children's perception of the experience. In assisting a family to resolve the negative feelings about a cesarean birth, health care providers should give the parents support and encouragement for discussing their feelings. If they are well-read in the field, they can also reflect the feelings of other parents to their patients.

INTERVIEWS WITH CESAREAN FAMILIES

To obtain an indication of how well children comprehend cesarean birth, we interviewed children in 9 families with from 2 to 4 children. In each family, at least one child had been born by cesarean. All parents of these children had the attitude toward cesarean birth that, "They would not choose it," but they did "accept its necessity." In other words, none of the children's parents harbored bitter, negative or depressed feelings over their cesareans. In 7 of the families the parents had given a thorough and clear explanation of cesarean birth. In two, the explanation was described as "minimal."

We asked each child to tell us what a cesarean birth is. Following are their answers:

Girl, age 5: "I don't know (what cesarean birth is)."

Girl, age 7: ''Mommy was put to sleep when my brother was born. We went up to visit her a lot. Sometimes the baby comes out from the stomach.''

Girl, age 8: ''A cesarean is when they have to cut open the stomach.''

Girl, age 10: ''(A cesarean is when) the baby is born in a way that it's too big to come out, so they cut open the stomach and they take the baby out of the uterus. It seems a little scary to have it done to you. I'd probably want it so that I could see, so I knew what was happening.''

Girl, age 10: ''She was going to have a vaginal birth but the baby was not in the right position, so she couldn't. So the doctor cut open the mother's stomach and took the baby out. I saw a movie of a cesarean birth on T.V. and it was kind of gross. The doctor had to reach in and take things out.''

Boy, age 6: ''You tell me (what a cesarean birth is). I don't know.

Boy, age 8: ''Cesarean birth? It's a hard question. The baby was pretty fat so she had to cut open her — what is it? — uterus, because it was too fat to go down her little tunnel.''

Boy, age 9: ''A cesarean is when they cut open your stomach and then they take the baby out. It's not any big deal — it's just different.''

Boy, age 9: ''A cesarean birth is when a baby is larger than usual and sometimes the mother has medical problems, they have to cut the mother's stomach and take the baby out.''

Most children, while curious about cesarean birth, do not dwell on it or spend much time thinking about it. A major reason for defining the process for the younger children is to include them in the general family experience. If they feel comfortable with the subject when they are young, they feel free to ask for more information when they want to know more.

THE FATHER'S ROLE

Cesarean birth offers fathers a unique opportunity to make things run smoothly at home, especially if there is an older child. In addition to participating in the explanation of the operation, the father can explain in advance to the child that the mother's abdomen will be tender so she won't be able to hold the child on her lap for a while. He can make plans with the child for them to enjoy some special occasions while the mother is in the hospital — go to a restaurant, visit the library and find books about babies, visit a favorite park. He can take the child to the hospital to visit the mother and baby and perhaps to have a meal with the mother in the hospital cafeteria.

116

The father can stage the homecoming for the child's benefit by carrying the baby into the house himself. This leaves the mother free to embrace the child and it relieves her of the responsibility for the baby until everyone is settled. He can suggest that the mother get right to bed to continue recuperating. He can help the child be part of the family group by having the child sit quietly near the mother on the bed before they leave her to rest.

At some point the father and the child can take the baby into another room to get acquainted. He can help the child learn to touch the baby's arms and legs and head while pointing out that the baby's face is too delicate to touch. He can encourage the child to chatter, sing and coo with the baby. These little events will be major ones for the child — they will help the child feel important to the baby and to the father while teaching the child how to act with the baby.

BIBLIOGRAPHY

Baker, Gayle Cunningham, *Special Delivery: A Book for Kids About Cesarean & Vaginal Birth,* Seattle: Chas. Franklin Press. 1981.

Caveney, Sylvia, *Inside Mom,* New York: St. Martin's Press. 1977.

Donovan, Bonnie, *The Cesarean Birth Experience,* Boston: Beacon. 1977.

Elkind, David, *A Sympathetic Understanding of the Child: Birth to Sixteen.* Boston: Allyn and Bacon, Inc. 1971.

Elkind, David, *Child Development and Education — A Piagetian Perspective,* New York: Oxford University Press. 1976.

Hausknecht, Richard, *Having a Cesarean Baby,* New York: Dutton. 1978.

Holland, Viki, *We Are Having a Baby,* New York: Charles Scribner's Sons. 1972.

Rey, Hans Augusto, *Curious George Takes a Job,* Boston: Houghton Mifflin Company. 1947.

Sobol, Harriett Langsam, *Jeff's Hospital Book,* New York: Henry Z. Walck, Inc. 1975.

AN AFTERWORD

Children at Birth:
The Gentle Revolution

DAVID STEWART

We hold these truths to be self evident, that all men, women, children, parents and professionals are created equal; that they are endowed by their creator with certain unalienable rights; that among these are life, liberty, the pursuit of happiness, the right to a safe, natural birth assisted by and in the company of those who love them, the right to be well nourished in their mothers' wombs, and the right to be breastfed.

—The NAPSAC Declaration of Independence.

The inclusion of children at birth is probably the most profound development in the childbirth reform movement yet. It will be through these children that the goals of improved safety, humanity, and family-centered maternity care, so long fought for by parents, will eventually be accomplished. I came to realize this by observing my own children in public school. We have five, all born at home, and in every case, the older children have always been present to witness the births of their younger siblings. All of them were born naturally and were breastfed.

Jonathan, our oldest, is now seventeen and was present for the births of his younger sister and three brothers. He is well liked in school and pretty smart. He has already won some academic recognition, as well as awards in essay, speaking and music contests. He was elected to the high school student council by his classmates. He doesn't talk about his birth experiences, but everyone in the school knows about them and occasionally kids him in a good natured way. He is fully accepted by his peers.

I have recently realized that Jonathan's quiet presence in that school has indelibly planted the idea in the minds of every student (as well as many teachers) that, perhaps, natural childbirth, home birth, and breastfeeding are something to consider. They cannot escape at least thinking about it.

Every girl in that school, when she becomes pregnant at some future time, is at least going to think about.alternatives to current obstetric practice. She won't be able to help it. After all, a respected classmate of hers was born at home naturally, and breastfed — and so were his brothers and sister.

I have come to understand that having siblings at birth is not just a "nice thing to do." It is a profoundly revolutionary thing to do in the truest sense of revolution. The enlightened childbirth movement will have achieved its goal when it becomes second nature for every pregnant woman to consider midwifery, natural childbirth, breastfeeding, etc., as being the normal choices in having a baby. Not only will the children who attend births do this themselves, so will their friends and contacts.

APPENDIX A

INTERVIEW PROTOCOL

I.   Family Activities in Preparation for the Baby.

Below is a list of activities parents might use to help children be prepared for the coming baby. Please answer yes, or no, if you used this activity.

A. Brought the children into your discussion about the baby?

Yes _____ No (don't approve) _____ No (didn't think of it) _____

What stimulated the discussion?

When in relation to expected date of birth?

B. Let the child/ren feel the baby move in your abdomen?

Yes _____ No (don't approve) _____ No (didn't think of it) _____

When?

Where?

How often?

Reaction of child/ren?

C. Brought the child/ren to prenatal visits?

Yes _____ No (don't approve) _____ No (didn't think of it) _____

How often?

Reaction?

D. Let the child/ren listen to fetal heart?

Yes _____ No (don't approve) _____ No (didn't think of it) _____

Reaction?

E. Showed the child/ren pictures of babies, and talked about them?

Yes ＿＿ No (don't approve) ＿＿ No (didn't think of it) ＿＿

F. Showed the child/ren the clothes and equipment for the baby?

Yes ＿＿ No (don't approve) ＿＿ No (didn't think of it) ＿＿

G. Let the child/ren handle the baby's things?

Yes ＿＿ No (don't approve) ＿＿ No (didn't think of it) ＿＿

H. Answered the child/ren's questions: Where is the baby? How did he get there? How will he get out? Etc.

Yes ＿＿ No (don't approve) ＿＿ No (didn't think of it) ＿＿

I. Let the child/ren try the things for the baby, such as diapers, baby bottle, baby's bed?

Yes ＿＿ No (don't approve) ＿＿ No (didn't think of it) ＿＿

J. Gave a small doll to the child/ren to be his/her baby?

Yes ＿＿ No (don't approve) ＿＿ No (didn't think of it) ＿＿

K. Brought child/ren to child birth preparation class(es)?

Yes ＿＿ No (don't approve) ＿＿ No (didn't think of it) ＿＿

Which group?

Child/ren's reaction?

L. To childbirth films?

Yes ＿＿ No (don't approve) ＿＿ No (didn't think of it) ＿＿

Which film?

Child/ren's reaction?

II. Reaction of Child/ren at the Birth.

   A. Where was the child/ren during labor and birth?

   B. Who related to child/ren during the birth?

   C. In what way did the child/ren participate in the birth?

   D. Overall reaction of child/ren to:
       Mother:

       Father:

       Other Siblings:

       Newborn:

III. Reaction of the Child/ren to the Baby during First Week.

   A. Wanted to hold baby.   Yes _____ No _____
   B. Wanted to participate in care.   Yes _____ No _____
   C. Wanted to comfort baby.   Yes _____ No _____
   D. Returned to baby talk.   Yes _____ No _____
   E. Returned to daytime wetting.   Yes _____ No _____
   F. Returned to nighttime wetting.   Yes _____ No _____
   G. Returned to thumb sucking.   Yes _____ No _____
   H. Wants to sleep in baby's crib.   Yes _____ No _____
   I. Wants to drink from the breast
       or bottle although off the
       bottle normally.   Yes _____ No _____
   J. Wants to wear diapers although
       normally does not wear them.   Yes _____ No _____
   K. Abuses or strikes the baby.   Yes _____ No _____
   L. Strikes you when you hold the baby.   Yes _____ No _____

III. Reaction of the children to the Baby during First Week (continued)

    M. Strikes your husband when he
       holds the baby.   Yes _____   No _____

    N. Tries to push baby off lap.   Yes _____   No _____

    O. Acting out in other ways when
       mother occupied with baby.   Yes _____   No _____

IV. Reaction of Child to Parents during First Week.

V. Long-term Relationship of Child and Infant.

VI. Has your child seen you undressed?

    _____ never

    _____ only in the bathroom

    _____ around the house

    _____ other situations

_____

_____

_____

APPENDIX B

PROJECT TITLE:
EFFECTS OF BIRTHS OF SIBLINGS ON CHILDREN

INTERVIEW FORM

Interview Number _____

I.   The birth (for children present)

  A. Do you remember your baby sister/brother being born?
      Tell me about it.

  B. Did you help at the birth?

      How?

  C. What did your Mom do when the baby was born?

  D. What did your Father do?

  E. What did the baby look like?

  F. Would you like to see another baby be born?

II. The birth (for children not present).

  A. What were you doing when your baby sister/brother was born?

  B. Did you visit your Mom in the hospital?
      Tell me about it.

  C. What did the baby look like?

124

II. The birth (for children not present) (continued)

D. Would you like to see a baby be born?

III. When you're older, do you think you will have children?

IV. Relationship to sibling.
A. Tell me how you get along with your baby sister/brother.

B. What do you like about her/him?

C. What don't you like about her/him?

V. Draw me a picture of a baby being born.
Tell me about it.

VI. Draw me a picture of your family.
Tell me about it.

APPENDIX C

SUMMARY OF SUGGESTIONS

The following list contains suggestions for the preparation of children for newborn siblings, for the facilitation of participation of children at birth, and the integration of children in the postpartum period. Many of the suggestions can be carried out by the parents in the home setting. There are also suggestions for childbirth educators and health professionals who are interested in incorporating siblings into the pregnancy, birth and postpartum period, being sensitive to the wishes of the children and parents.

The breadth and depth of the preparation and support needed and wanted by children depends on their ages, level of development, and interests. Each child will benefit most by individually styled responses. However, it is possible to carry out some of the preparation in small groups.

Most of the suggestions are appropriate for the home, birth center or hospital setting. Adaptations will depend on the resources in the environment and the creativity of support persons and children, parents and staff. A support person should always be present for each child in any setting, but the younger child will undoubtedly require the most supervision and support.

These suggestions are listed in a brief form. For more information please see the chapters in the book, and list of educational resources in Appendix D.

SUGGESTIONS FOR PARENTS

I. To prepare child to be present at birth of sibling

    A. Early discussion with child on following topics:
- expanding family
- conception and sexuality; the human body
- feelings and fantasies about birth and babies
- fetal development

    B. Include child in some prenatal exams
- to meet the doctor or midwife
- to listen to the fetal heart beat
- to feel the baby move
- to become used to physical exam of the mother's body

    C. Do prenatal exercises together with child.

    D. Read books to child about birth:
- pictures of fetal development
- Mom and Dad and I are Having a Baby
- Gabriel's Very First Birthday
- look at the child's own baby book and baby pictures

E. Take child to some prenatal classes to see films, videotapes, slides, and posters, preferably in color. Tour of birthing room.

F. Demonstrate birth with dolls, puppets.

G. Have child draw pictures of a baby being born and of the family.

H. Familiarize child with the following:
— equipment for birth in home or hospital and things not to touch
— sounds of labor, the intensity, pain and hard work
— wetness of birth, the blood and bag of waters
— painless cutting of cord, like cutting hair
— appearance and capabilities of newborn
— placenta
— method of feeding baby

I. Inform child of duties of mother, father, midwife/doctor, and support person, so child knows the parents will be busy, but that someone will be there just for him or her.

J. Explain possible alterations in the birth plan:
— unknown length of labor and birth
— child might be sleeping or at school
— need for mother to be transported to hospital, delivery room, or surgery
— need for baby to be taken care of by doctors if baby is sick
— needs of mother for privacy, quiet and rest
— possible interventions, e.g., episiotomy

II. To facilitate participation of child at birth

A. A special person, such as grandparent, babysitter, friend or neighbor to be with child all the time, including the postpartum period. It is ideal if this person attends classes with child and tours the birthing room.

B. Freedom of movement for child in and out of the birth setting.

C. Recognition of child by parents between contractions.

D. Provide tasks for child:
— bringing cool cloths
— bringing something for mother to drink
— massage
— walking with mother
— changing phonograph records; photography

E. Special or favorite toys or projects that can be done quietly:
— books, puzzles, games, dolls, cards

F. Comfort measures for child:
    — sleeping bag, blanket
    — snacks, juice

G. Supervised interaction with newborn:
    — touching, massaging, holding
    — Leboyer bath
    — giving a gift

H. If child was not present at birth, provide opportunity for togetherness in recovery room.

I. Family celebration with birthday cake, gifts, and appropriate family rituals.

III. To integrate children in postpartum period

A. Space for child and accompanying adult in waiting room. Child should not be left unattended.

B. Acquaint child with rules of hospital, e.g., quiet, no running, no playing in the elevators.

C. Contact with mother and newborn, following possible hospital rules for hand-washing and gowning.

D. Provide books for children about living with a baby:
    — Our Brand New Baby
    — On Mother's Lap

E. Tell child of special needs of mother for quiet and rest.

F. Include child in care of baby as appropriate:
    — changing diapers
    — feeding baby
    — tasting breast milk if child is curious
    — bathing

G. Debriefing of child in days following birth:
    — drawing pictures of the birth
    — writing a story
    — sharing news with other family and friends
    — reliving birth by rereading books on birth, playing with birthing doll, and looking at child's own baby pictures.

SUGGESTIONS FOR CHILDBIRTH EDUCATORS/ HEALTH PROFESSIONALS

I. Inform parents of various ways child can be included in pregnancy, birth, and postpartum period.

II. Include decisions about sibling participation in birth plan, their ages and interests.

III. Suggest to parents ways to prepare children. If possible, meet with child one to three times before the birth:
   A. Read books to child.
   B. Simulate labor.
   C. Play with birthing dolls.
   D. View slides, providing age-appropriate explanations and engaging the child in dialogue.
   E. Draw pictures and tell stories about drawings.
   F. Desensitization to blood, e.g., in books and slides, viewing placenta. If child chooses, he or she can use gloves to touch placenta and see how blood fills the vessels.

IV. Tour of birth room with introduction to equipment.

V. Acquaint support person with hospital environment:
   — waiting room and bathroom
   — cafeteria and outdoor areas
   — nearby restaurants, parks, libraries

VI. Provide information on parenting and books to be read to children in the days following the birth.

APPENDIX D

EDUCATIONAL RESOURCES FOR "EXPECTING" SIBLINGS

Audio-Visuals:

BREASTFEEDING — A FAMILY EVENT, slide show with cassette tape and instructor's guide, $50. Bay Area ASPO Slides. c/o Deanna Sollid, R.N., 59 Berens Drive, Kentfield, CA 94904. Shows the emotional and physical preparation of the expectant parents for breastfeeding, as well as the development of the nursing relationship, helping a sibling to adjust and the importance of the husband's supportive role.

SIBLINGS AND BIRTH, color slide series with teaching index showing sibling preparation, participation and bonding as well as aspects of labor, birth and newborn appearance that are important elements in preparing siblings who will participate in birth. 74 color slides, $35 + $3.50 postage and handling. Preview sheet available upon request. Childbirth Graphics, PO Box 17025, Irondequoit, Rochester, NY 14617.

ANTHONY'S BIRTH AT HOME. When the woman in this film was expecting her first child she could not find a medical attendant who would come to her home for her labor and delivery. She and her husband decided to have the baby at home without medical supervision with the husband attending. This film tells the story of Anthony, their fifth child, born at home, delivered by his father.

"Anthony's Birth at Home" is a 16mm color/sound film with a running time of 17 minutes. Cinema Medica, 664 N. Michigan Ave., Chicago, IL. 60611.

Purchase: 16mm $265
          Super 8 Cartridge $250
          Video Cassette $250
Rental: $35

BIRTH CENTERS. To combat the trend to home births and to avoid the dehumanization of the labor and delivery room technology, birth centers have opened in and out of the hospitals around the country. In this film you will see and hear parents and professionals give their views on birth centers and you will see couples giving birth in them.

"Birth Centers" is a 16mm color/sound film with a running time of 24 minutes. Cinema Medica, 664 N. Michigan Ave., Chicago, IL. 60611.

Purchase: 16mm $295
         Super 8 Cartridge $250
         Video Cassette $250
Rental: $35

CHILDREN AT BIRTH. From the hatching of chickens to the birth of a baby and the delivery of the placenta, this very gentle film prepares children of any age for the miracle of birth. Children are present at their siblings' births which occur both in and out of the hospital setting.

"Children at Birth" is a 16mm color/sound film with a running time of 24 minutes. Cinema Medica, 664 N. Michigan Ave., Chicago, IL. 60611.

Purchase: 16mm $295
         Super 8 Cartridge $250
         Video Cassette $250
Rental: $35

TAMIKA'S BIRTH. The film features an overview of pregnancy, birth, and the postpartum period. The story of Tamika's birth portrays a black family's experience during pregnancy and the birth of a new baby.

Childbirth Education Films, Videograph, 2833 25th Street, San Francisco, CA. 94110. 11-minute, color 16mm film and ¾ " videocassette.

Purchase: $185
Rental: $25

THE WELCOMING: A FAMILY BIRTH EXPERIENCE. This is the story of how a 3½ yr. old child was prepared to view and participate in the birth, and her reaction to it.

The slides show an unmedicated birth, bonding, warm water bath, and the welcoming of a new baby into a family.

"The Welcoming: A Family Birth Experience," L. Wermuth, R.N., 1979. Show and Tell Instructional Aides, 2905 Cambridge Drive, San Jose, CA. 95125. 33mm color slides and cassette tape gives guidelines for training children who expect to be present at the birth of a sibling. This film is suitable for viewing by childbirth educators, expectant parents, children, and professionals concerned with natural childbirth.

NICHOLAS AND THE BABY. Through the humor and warmth of the child's perspective, this unique film provides a gentle way of introducing parents to the perceptions and questions of children and introducing children from 4 to 12 to the facts and feelings involved with the birth of a sibling. Enhanced by an animated sequence on fetal development, the music of Carl Orff, and a detailed Parent/Teacher Study Guide, "Nicholas and the

Baby'' sensitively portrays all the excitement and drama of a family-oriented pregnancy, labor and birth.

The birth includes the use of fetal monitor, intravenous feeding, and transfer to the delivery room. Nicholas is not present for the birth, but meets his sister soon after and celebrates the ''birthday party'' with the family in the hospital.

''Nicholas and the Baby'' is a 16mm film with a running time of 23 minutes. Centre Productions Inc., 1312 Pine St., Suite A, Boulder, CO. 80302.

Purchase: 16 mm $350
           ¾ Video Cassette $275
Rental: $35 (plus $7.00 for shipping & handling)

Books:

Andry, A.C., *Hi, New Baby*. NY: Simon and Schuster, 1970.

Andry, A.C. and Scheff, S., *How Babies Are Made*. NY: Time-Life Books, 1968. Straightforward presentation of reproduction of flowers, chickens, dogs and humans. Paper sculpture illustrations.

Berenstain, S. and Berenstain, J., *The Berenstain Bears' New Baby*. NY: Random House, 1974.

Brown, J., Lesser, E., Mines, S., Buryn, E., *Two Births*. Berkeley, CA: Random House, 1972.

Caveney, S., *Inside Mom*. NY: St. Martins Press, 1977. Information about the developing fetus and changes taking place during pregnancy.

Dragonwagon, C., *Wind Rose*. NY: Harper and Row, 1976. A mother tells her daughter just what she and daddy felt, dreamed and planned while waiting for her to be born. Drawings and text describe the home birth itself.

Faison, E. and Ergin, C., *Becoming*. Waitsfield, VT: Vermont Crossroads Press, 1976.

Farrell, S., *Gabriel's Very First Birthday*. Seattle, WA: Pipeline Books, 1976. Photos and text tell about the home birth of Gabriel. *Out of Print*.

Gruenberg, S., *The Wonderful Story of How You Were Born*. NY: Doubleday, 1970.

Hathaway, M. and Hathaway, J., *Children at Birth*. Sherman Oaks, CA: Academy Publications, 1978. Presents a positive case for having children present at siblings' births. Explores pros and cons and contains reports from children themselves. Over 125 photos.

132

Kaefring, G., *Mama Gives Birth Coloring Book*. Iowa City, IA: Emma Goldman Clinic for Women, 1978.

Malecki, M., *Mom and Dad and I Are Having a Baby*. Seattle, WA: Pennypress, 1979. The purpose of this book is to prepare children who will be present for the birth of a sibling. The experience of the author, who is a mother, childbirth educator, nurse and birth attendant, has been that most children are "inadequately prepared for the sights and sounds of birth." In hopes of decreasing this lack of preparation of children, "this book is designed so that it can be enjoyed and understood by children of all ages. For older children, the complete text on the left page may be read by the parents. For the young child the pictures and captions will tell the story."

The book includes accurate information and realistic pencil drawings, with an emphasis on the things that are most upsetting to children: hurting of mother, loud noises of pushing, blood, umbilical cord, placenta, appearance of newborn, and cutting the cord. Some of the attractive illustrations have been highlighted with color in order to use visual communication in addition to the written text to clarify the scenes that seem to have the most emotional impact on the child; for instance, the placenta is purple, the face of the pushing mother is red, the newborn and cord are greyish-blue, and several drawings clearly show the presence of blood.

Malecki, M., *Our Brand New Baby*. Seattle, WA: Pennypress, 1980. This book is a sequel to the above, preparing the older child for life with a new baby.

Nilsson, L. et al., *A Child Is Born*. NY: Delacorte Press, 1977.

Nilsson, L., *How Was I Born?* NY: Delacorte Press, 1975. Story of reproduction and birth for children.

Rogers, F., *Mister Rogers Talks about the New Baby*. NY: Platt and Munk, 1974.

Rushnell, E., *My Mom's Having a Baby*. NY: Grosset and Dunlap, 1978. Based on the ABC television presentation, including a hospital birth.

Scott, A., *On Mother's Lap*. NY: McGraw-Hill, 1972. A young Eskimo boy discovers that even with a new baby, there is still room for him.

Scott, L. and Baze, D., *My Childbirth Coloring Book*. Chicago, IL: Academy Press Ltd., 1978. Story told by child as narrator whose sex is not apparent. May be used for any age child. Natural facts of life explained so information can be received on many levels.

Sheffield, M., *Where Do Babies Come From?* NY: Alfred Knopf, 1973. Honestly answers the question in the text and pastel paintings.

Sinberg, J., *We Got This New Baby at Our House.* NY: Avon Books, 1980.

Showers, P., *A Baby Starts to Grow.* NY: Thomas Y. Crowell, 1969.

Showers, P. and Showers, K., *Before You Were a Baby.* NY: Thomas Y. Crowell, 1968.

Waxman, S., *What Is a Girl? What Is a Boy?* Culver City, CA: Peace Press, 1976. Simple logical text discusses issue of sexual identity. Includes children's drawings and photographs of male and female bodies.

Young, F., *Gerald the Third.* La Leche League, 1977. Story of one six-year-old's family, including the birth of a younger sister. Written to stimulate discussion with children about family life, feedings and attitudes.

Magazines:

"Birth" in *Children's Express,* Special Edition, International Year of the Child, Children's Cultural Foundation, Inc., 66 Bank St., New York, NY 10014.

Teaching Aids/Toys:

FETAL MODELS: Soft flexible cloth body with firm "molded" head, approximately newborn size. Useful in demonstrating many aspects of labor and birth. Also available are a detachable placenta and cord and knitted uterus and vagina. All are available in kit or completed form from Childbirth Graphics, PO Box 17025. Irondequoit, Rochester, NY 14617.

NATALIE, a 22 inch birthing rag doll, and BERTHA RAGS, a 19 inch birthing monkey doll with detachable cords and placentas. Adaptable for cesarean birth. Monkey Business, Box 2603, Tallahassee, FL 32304.

AUTHOR INDEX

SUBJECT INDEX